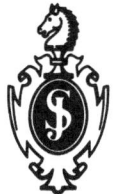

Nigel Kirkham, Dennis W.K. Cotton,
Roger C. Lallemand, John E. White
and R. David Rosin (Eds.)

Diagnosis and Management of Melanoma in Clinical Practice

With 70 Figures

Springer-Verlag London Ltd.

Nigel Kirkham, Consultant Pathologist
Royal Sussex County Hospital, Brighton
BN2 5BE

Roger C. Lallemand, Consultant Surgeon
Frimley Park Hospital, Frimley, Surrey

R. David Rosin, Consultant Surgeon 6
Harley Street, London W1N 1AA

Dennis W.K. Cotton, Senior Lecturer
Department of Pathology, The University
of Sheffield, PO Box 596, Sheffield
S10 2UL

John E. White, Consultant Dermatologist
Royal South Hants Hospital,
Southampton SO9 4PE

Cover illustration: Clinical photographs with kind permission of Dr Nigel Kirkham;
Fig. 7.9 reproduced from Smith (1987), with kind permission.

British Library Cataloguing in Publication Data
Diagnosis and management of melanoma in clinical practice
I. Title
616.994075

Library of Congress Cataloging-in-Publication Data
Diagnosis and management of melanoma in clinical practice/Kirkham ... (et al.).
  p. cm.
Includes index.
ISBN 978-1-4471-1927-2   ISBN 978-1-4471-1925-8 (eBook)
DOI 10.1007/978-1-4471-1925-8

1. Melanoma.I. Kirkham, Nigel, 1952–
[DNLM: 1. Melanoma–diagnosis. 2. Melanoma–therapy.   QZ 200 D5368]
RC280.M37D53 1992
616.99'477–dc20
DNLM/DLC   91-5135
for Library of Congress   CIP

Typeset by Wilmaset, Birkenhead, Wirral

2128/3830-543210 Printed on acid-free paper

*This book is dedicated to the memory of
Brian Macdougall.*

Preface

Melanoma presents a problem with many faces. It is a malignancy that kills many young people and once established is very refractory to treatment. It is most effectively managed by primary prevention or by early recognition and excision. We look to oncologists and pigment cell biologists to find possible new avenues for effective therapies.

The Melanoma Study Group has provided a forum in Britain for the presentation and discussion of developments in the field. The Group has always fostered a multidisciplinary approach and is pleased to be able to present this collection of reviews of current problems and advances.

The book has been compiled by inviting contributions from a wide range of authors each of whom is actively involved in the area they describe. The epidemiology of melanoma continues to advance, with some early evidence that the message of prevention may at last be having an effect in slowing the previously unstoppable increase in prevalence seen in the West. The problems of the clinical recognition of pigmented lesions are dealt with by an illustrated guide to differential diagnoses; by a demonstration of the way that algorithms can aid in structuring the way we make our differential diagnoses; and by a presentation of the potential that computed image analysis has for screening and early diagnosis of melanoma.

The continuing debate about familial melanoma and dysplastic naevi is viewed from a clinical perspective, with pointers to a pragmatic solution to these problems. The histopathology and criteria for diagnosis of melanoma is a constant problem especially where borderline lesions are concerned. The book includes contributions that discuss the diagnosis of malignant lesions and that point out benign lesions that may be mistaken for melanoma.

Further chapters present reviews of prognostic factors; the surgical approach to the disease in all of its stages; the place for isolated limb perfusion; the methods of systemic chemotherapy most likely to produce results; and the prospects for specific therapeutic targeting of disseminated melanoma. Finally, when all else has failed we are still left with the fears and concerns of the individual patient. A review of issues in counselling melanoma patients addresses these problems.

This book will be essential reading for anybody involved in the study or management of melanoma. Specialists in dermatology, general and plastic surgery, oncology, histopathology and epidemiology will find new information in their own field and understandable reviews of other specialties. General practitioners, who are involved in the early detection of melanoma and the management and counselling of those with established disease, will also find much to interest them.

Brighton   Nigel Kirkham
September 1991   Dennis W.K. Cotton
                                                                                  Roger C. Lallemand
                                                                                          John E. White
                                                                                  R. David Rosin

Contents

Contributors

R.E. Ashton
Consultant Dermatologist, Department of Dermatology, Royal
Naval Hospital, Haslar, Gosport, Hants PO12 2AA

Michele M. Delaunay
Consultant Dermatologist, Chr Pellegrin, Place Amelie Rabat
Leon, F-33000 Bordeaux, France

Judy Evans
Consultant Plastic Surgeon, Department of Plastic Surgery,
Derriford Hospital, Plymouth, Devon PL6 8DH

Lesley Fallowfield
Senior Lecturer in Health Psychology, The London Hospital
Medical College, 3rd Floor Alexandra Wing, Turner Street,
London E1 2AD

P. Hall
Research Registrar in Plastic Surgery, The Queen Victoria
Hospital, Holtye Road, East Grinstead, West Sussex RH19 3DZ

B.W. Hancock
Professor of Clinical Oncology, Weston Park Hospital, Sheffield
S10 2SJ

T. Krausz
Consultant Histopathologist, Royal Postgraduate Medical School,
Hammersmith Hospital, Du Cane Road, London W12 0NN

J.A.H. Lee
Department of Epidemiology SC-36, School of Public Health,
University of Washington, Seattle, Washington 98195, USA

Rona M. MacKie
Professor of Dermatology, Department of Dermatology, Anderson
College Building, 56 Dumbarton Road, Glasgow G11 6NU

W.J. Mooi
Head of Department of Pathology, The Netherlands Cancer
Institute, Antoni van Leeuwenhoek Huis, Plesmanlaan 121, 1066
CX Amsterdam, The Netherlands

Julia A. Newton
Consultant Dermatologist, Department of Dermatology, Royal
London Hospital, Whitechapel, London E1 1BB

P.A. Riley
Professor of Cell Pathology, Department of Chemical Pathology,
University College and Middlesex School of Medicine, Cleveland
Street, London W1P 6DB

R.D. Rosin
Consultant Surgeon, 6 Harley Street, London W1N 1AA

E. Sheridan
Clinical Research Fellow, Weston Park Hospital, Sheffield S10 2SJ

N.P. Smith
Consultant Dermatologist, St John's Dermatology Centre, St
Thomas's Hospital, Lambeth Palace Road, London SE1 7EH

1   Epidemiology of Malignant Melanoma

J. A. H. Lee

Complexity and Dissonance

The melanomas occur at a variety of anatomical sites, different phenotypes and genotypes strongly influence their incidence, and they have recognizable precursor lesions. All of this variation presents opportunities for fruitful comparisons. As a result, in a high risk population known factors can account for perhaps half the cases (English and Armstrong 1988). This is about the same as the proportion for female breast cancer (Bruzzi et al. 1985). Yet the epidemiology of melanoma is loaded with paradox. Generalizations, if they can be offered at all, are hedged with exceptions. New data, for example the finding that in a high risk population, small melanomas were not associated with the usual host factors (Schneider et al. 1987), often do not fit in.

It is not clear whether this is an expression of the complexity of the neoplastic changes of the melanocyte, or merely that our level of information is adequate for confusion but not yet for synthesis. Either way, the current difficulties present researchable problems. The following notes draw attention to a few of these. Each in some way does not fit into current ideas, and each is an unexpected finding or has resisted enquiry. Some have been known about for years, whereas others are recent.

The following is not a comprehensive summary of modern knowledge of the epidemiology of melanoma. The older literature is thoroughly surveyed in Longstreth (1987). A number of excellent recent shorter accounts are readily available (Evans et al. 1988; Osterlind 1990).

Recall Bias

Much of the causation of melanoma is related to the things people do, and the reaction of their bodies to this. Prospective studies of what is still a fairly rare

Table 1.1. Ability to tan, as reported before diagnosis of melanoma and afterwards. Modified from Nurses Health Study (1976–84) (Weinstock et al. 1991)

	Before diagnosis	After diagnosis	Percentage change
No tan, or light tan	9	15	66.67
Average tan	18	17	− 5.56
Deep tan	7	2	−71.43
Total	34	34	

disease must be prohibitively large to obtain results, and the usual approach is to gather data on behaviour and physical reaction by asking questions of people with the disease and comparing the answers with those from people without. In a recent large prospective study of many aspects of the health of nurses, 34 of them developed melanomas over the years. They were asked about their ability to tan, and the answers were compared with the responses the same women gave long before their diagnosis (Table 1.1) (Weinstock et al. 1991). There was a substantial, and statistically significant, shift towards a reported low ability to tan. In contrast, the respondents gave similar answers before and after diagnosis to a question about their natural hair colour. A study comparing cases and controls would have exaggerated the importance of the tanning reaction. This finding was a surprise, as there are many areas where a diagnosis does not change memories. Contemporary estimates of the importance of, for example, severe sunburns in melanoma aetiology become questionable.

Exposure

The relationship of melanoma incidence to phenotype, and to latitude of residence, and its rapid secular change all indicate the importance of exposure. However, outdoor work substantially reduces melanoma risk, and indeed, the decline in outdoor jobs over recent decades has been suggested as contributing to the rising incidence of melanoma (Gallagher et al. 1987, 1989).

The effects of severe exposure can be quite modest. For example, vacations spent by Danes on Mediterranean beaches only increased their melanoma risk by about 40% (Osterlind et al. 1988a) (Table 1.2). In contrast, in the same study, the

Table 1.2. Vacations in Southern Europe or similar sunny places and melanoma risk, Denmark, 1982–85. (From Osterlind et al. 1988a)

Vacation	Population	Relative risk	Relative risk (adjusted for sunbathing and sunburn)
Never	39%	1.0	1.0
Sunny resorts (sun + culture)	48%	1.2	1.0
Very sunny resorts (sun only)	13%	1.7	1.4

Table 1.3. Levels of reported sun exposure in childhood and youth by reported tanning ability. Control subjects without disease; sexes combined; western Washington, 1984–87. (Personal communication, Dr C.S. Kirkpatrick)

Sun exposure	No tan/mild tan/freckles		Moderate tan/deep tan		Percentage change between reported phenotypes
	No. of subjects	Percentage	No. of subjects	Percentage	
Age 2–10 years					
Low	46	65.71	102	52.04	72
Med	22	31.43	87	44.39	182
High	2	2.86	7	3.57	127
All	70	100.00	196	100.00	100
Age 11–20 years					
Low	53	73.61	105	53.30	72
Med	17	23.61	85	43.15	183
High	2	2.78	7	3.55	128
All	72	100.00	197	100.00	100

daily difference in exposure produced by men wearing trousers and women skirts produced a fivefold excess for the female leg (Osterlind et al. 1988b).

Subjects without skin disease should give reasonably unbiased histories of sun exposure. Data from control subjects selected at random from the population exemplify this (Table 1.3). They show, as would be expected, that persons who do not tan well recollect less sun exposure as children than persons who do. This is not surprising, but it illustrates the importance of baseline information in the evaluation of educational programmes.

Sex and Prognosis

It has been realized from clinical experience for many years that females with melanoma have a better prognosis than males. The difference persists for pre- and postmenopausal females, and seems independent of anatomical site. In several large-scale and careful studies, pregnancy was found to be irrelevant. A recent large-scale and meticulously conducted study of the Finnish cancer registry data (Karjalainen and Hakulinen 1988) ended with the conclusion: "The results indicate that a difference in patient's delay between males and females could be of importance in explaining the female superiority in survival. Some biological features related to sex itself might also have a significant effect on survival." These ideas have been expressed many times before. There is a clear need for some new variable to be measured, perhaps related to the extra female X chromosome, and the two sets of alleles for the genes on it. Or, we need to ask better questions about disease perception and care seeking.

Age and the Neoplastic Process

The low mean age at which melanoma is diagnosed or causes death compared with tumours of, for example, the colon, is an artefact of the cohort differences. The incidence of melanoma within the same group of people really increases steadily with age, just like an ordinary carcinoma. Naevi – common or dysplastic – decline in prevalence with increasing age (Nordlund et al. 1985). Declining prevalence of precursor lesions ought to limit the rise with age. Perhaps in the nevi that are going to produce melanomas, the damage is done early and they are immortalized? Or perhaps the immune system is better capable of coping in the young. In patients who suffered recurrent disease, the interval between primary treatment and recurrence was related to initial tumour thickness (Schultz et al. 1990). This interval was shorter in patients over 50 years than in younger patients. As might be expected from the earlier studies showing that the female advantage in prognosis was independent of age (Karjalainen and Hakulinen 1988), this age-related tumour progression was similar in males and females.

Rising Incidence Rates

General agreement has developed that the incidence rate for malignant mela-noma of the skin is rising rapidly among the prosperous white populations of the world (Muir and Neetoux 1982; Roush et al. 1985; Osterlind et al. 1988c). Numerous studies have found that the changes in diagnostic criteria are of little importance (van der Esch et al. 1991).

In most populations the rise is greatest for the male trunk, then for the limbs, in both sexes. There has been little change in rates for the head and neck. Interestingly, the rates for the melanomas of the choroidal tract of the eye have also remained approximately constant (Strickland and Lee 1981; Osterlind 1987). Whether this is because the eye shares to some extent the exposures of the skin of the head and neck, or because of some deeper reason, is unknown.

Because so many are treated in doctor's offices and do not come to pathological examination, there are fewer data on the incidence of the non-melanoma skin cancers and their trend. However, it does appear that the incidence of these tumours is also rising rapidly (Glass and Hoover 1989; Gallagher et al. 1990).

Rising Population Death Rates

Survival from malignant melanoma has increased very markedly in recent years (Thorn et al. 1989), with cases being treated at a progressively earlier pathologi-cal stage (Drzewiecki et al. 1990). Thus the death rate is rising more slowly than the incidence rate. The mortality from malignant melanoma in whites for all ages

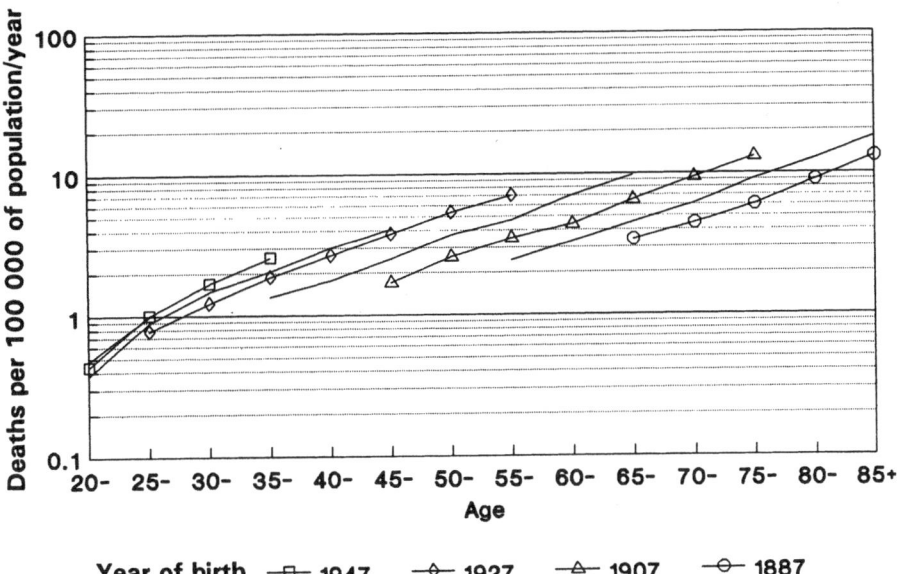

Fig. 1.1. US white male mortality from malignant melanoma of the skin by age for selected time periods, 1950–84.

in the United States increased, after age adjustment, over the period 1950–84 at about 3% a year in males and 2% in females. A number of studies have suggested that the disease is approaching its peak (Holman et al. 1980; Venzon and Moolgavkar 1984). A cohort diagram based on the US white male mortality data is given in Fig. 1.1. Apart from mathematical consideration, the development of naevi in childhood and youth, and the small extra risk run by adult migrants to sunny places, provides biological support for the idea that the levels of melanoma risk are determined in early life. The data on time trends have been reviewed recently (Lee 1991).

If the mortality data for the period 1950–84 are expressed as percentage changes for the separate age groups, they are found to vary markedly and systematically with age (Fig. 1.2). The largest increases were in the middle aged and old. The change over the time interval became progressively smaller in the younger groups, until it was actually negative in the youngest (Scotto et al. 1991). These differences in the age-specific behaviour of melanoma mortality are highly statistically significant. They clearly underlie the promise of stability in melanoma rates described by earlier authors, and in fact support projections of substantial declines in rates in the coming decades.

The explanation of the initial rising trend for malignant melanoma, and then, in particular age groups, its apparent decline, is not obvious. It is difficult to imagine progressive changes in the delivery of medical care that would have such a systematic relationship to age. The disease is more rapidly progressive in older persons (Schultz et al. 1990), so that the results of a general improvement in care might have a relationship to age imposed on them. Diagnosis is clearly getting earlier, but Scotto et al. (1991) were of the opinion that the limited incidence data indicated a pattern similar to the mortality data. If this is borne out by later

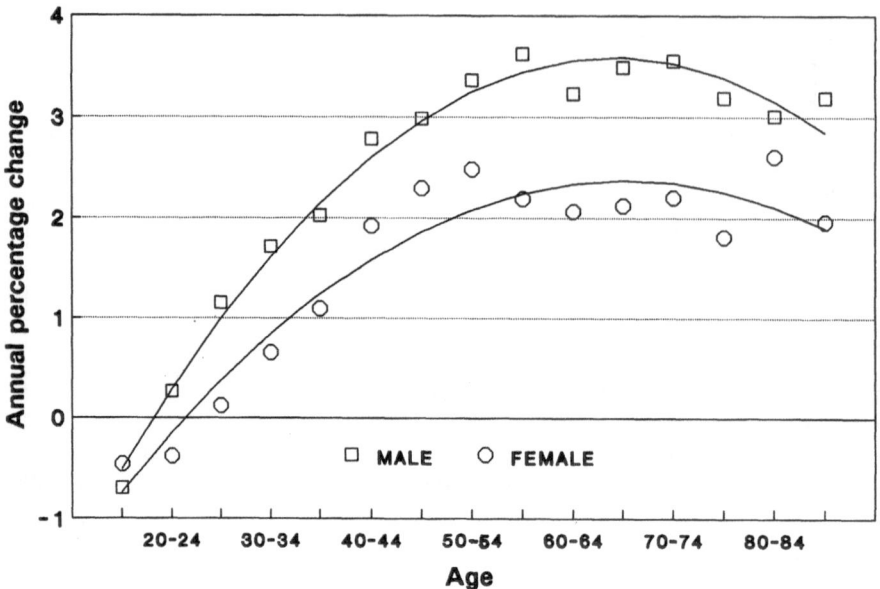

Fig. 1.2. Mean annual age-specific percentage change in mortality from malignant melanoma of the skin, 1950–84, US white males and females.

observations, it will suggest that the recent changes are being driven by the actual biology of the disease, rather than by its diagnosis.

The Ozone Layer

The association between increased melanoma risk and lack of pigmentation, which is similar to that found for the non-melanoma skin cancers, and the latitude gradients of risk within homogeneous populations underlines the relationship between the levels of melanoma risk in populations and exposure to sunlight. In the absence of an animal model for melanoma causation, the relative contribution of the different wavelengths in the solar spectrum is uncertain. However, the similarity of action spectra determined for a wide variety of biological effects suggests that the damage is largely done by the short UVB radiation around 300 nm.

In the Earth's upper atmosphere, there is a layer of ozone. This cuts off solar radiation at 295 nm. Many tonnes of chemically and biologically inert chlorofluorocarbon compounds have been, and continue to be, released to accumulate in the atmosphere. However, under the influence of the energetic solar radiation in the stratosphere, these molecules break up and release chlorine. This catalyses the destruction of ozone (Cicerone 1987). This analysis is not controversial (in contrast to the arguments about the heat-reflecting properties of carbon dioxide and other gases in the atmosphere). Up to the end of the 1980s, it was thought that although a decay in the ozone layer was measurable, it was not sufficient to cause biological effects (Scotto et al. 1987; Frederick et al. 1989). At the time useful, but limited, efforts were made to curb chlorofluorocarbon release. The Antarctic "ozone hole" is restricted in time and space, although its expression in 1990 was the biggest yet.

The most recent observations suggest that previous analyses were too optimistic (Green 1978; Reilly 1991), and that, apart from anything in Antarctica, a serious general decay in the ozone layer is in prospect. Substantial changes that are certain to have biological effects are predictable within a decade. It is particularly important to establish a sound basis from today's data for estimating future trends, as these will necessarily provide a standard by which the effects of future man-made changes in the intensity of sunlight will be judged.

Prognosis as Function of Incidence

The combination in Australia of high melanoma rates with high survival is well known. This may be a general relationship. Fig. 1.3 shows the survival as a function of incidence for the United States NCI SEER sites. The lines have been fitted to the data for the sites within the contiguous United States; the rates for Hawaiian whites are clearly different. It does not seem likely that the gradient in the United States could have been produced by an underlying gradient in public and professional awareness, and it may be that there is a biological relationship

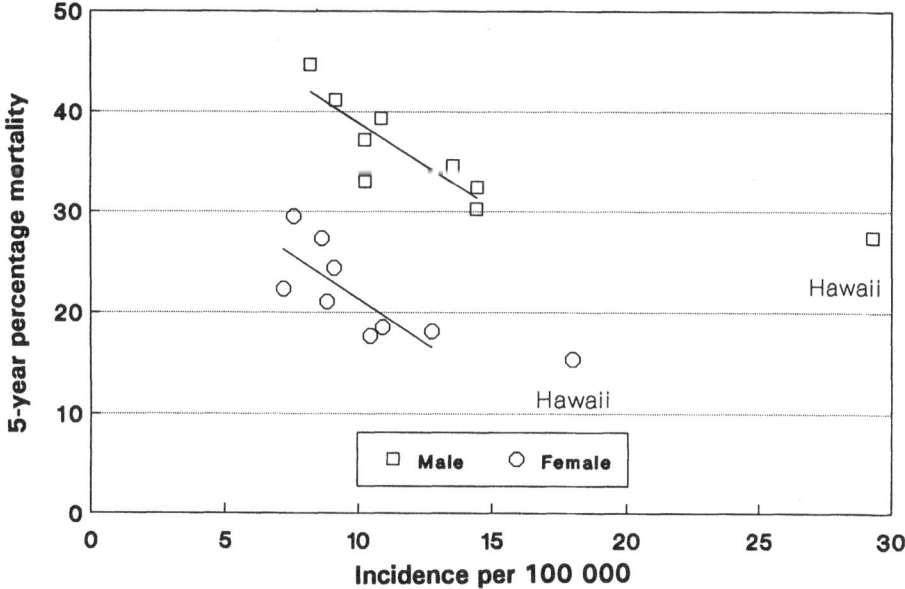

Fig. 1.3. Percentage mortality in five years from diagnosis by incidence of melanoma in the population. SEER areas of population-based cancer registration, 1974–84, by sex. The dependence of fatality on incidence is unlikely to be due to chance, both for all the SEER areas and for the contiguous US.

between incidence and survival (Lemish et al. 1983). A similar relationship between incidence and prognosis has been reported from Sweden (Lindegard 1990).

These data suggest that, as the ozone layer decays and presumably melanoma rates increase, the prognosis will also improve. Thus the consequences for mortality may be somewhat less than direct extrapolations would suggest. If the UV environment of Connecticut comes to approximate that prevailing in Georgia today, the inhabitants might expect many more melanomas, with an improvement in prognosis, but this will still lead to an increase in mortality. How these changes would interact with the temporal changes in the disease (Fig. 1.2) that have been going on for a long time is hard to estimate.

Conclusion

Variation between cases of a disease, between the incidence in different geographic populations, and between the risks for different kinds of people, often allow the development of fruitful hypotheses. These examples of the lack of congruence between different items of knowledge about the melanomas are offered with the hope that testable explanations will occur to people who are experts in other aspects of pigment cell biology, and who may not ordinarily have seen these epidemiological data.

References

Bruzzi P, Green SB, Byar DP, Brinton LA, Schairer C (1985) Estimating the population attributable risk for multiple risk factors using case-control data. Am J Epidemiol 122:904–914

Cicerone RJ (1987) Changes in stratospheric ozone. Science 237:35–42

Drzewiecki KT, Frydman H, Andersen PK, Poulsen H, Ladefoged C, Vibe P (1990) Malignant melanoma. Changing trends in factors influencing metastasis-free survival from 1964 to 1982. Cancer 65:362–366

English DR, Armstrong BK (1988) Identifying people at high risk of cutaneous malignant melanoma: results from a case-control study in Western Australia. Br Med J 296:1285–1288

Evans RD, Kopf AW, Lew RA et al. (1988) Risk factors for the development of malignant melanoma – 1: Review of case-control studies. Dermatol Surg Oncol 14:393–408

Frederick JE, Snell HE, Haywood EK (1989) Solar ultraviolet radiation at the earth's surface. Photochem Photobiol 50:443–450

Gallagher RP, Elwood JM, Threlfall WJ et al. (1987) Socioeconomic status, sunlight exposure, and risk of malignant melanoma: the Western Canada Melanoma Study. J Natl Cancer Inst 79:647–652

Gallagher RP, Elwood JM, Yang CP (1989) Is chronic sunlight exposure important in accounting for increases in melanoma incidence? Int J Cancer 44:813–815

Gallagher RP, Ma B, McLean DI et al. (1990) Trends in basal cell carcinoma, squamous cell carcinoma, and melanoma of the skin from 1973 through 1987. J Am Acad Dermatol 23:413–421

Glass AG, Hoover RN (1989) The emerging epidemic of melanoma and squamous cell cancer. JAMA 262:2097–2100

Green AES (1978) Ultraviolet exposure and skin cancer response. Am J Epidemiol 107:277–280

Holman CDJ, James IR, Gattey PH, Armstrong BK (1980) An analysis of trends in mortality from malignant melanoma of the skin in Australia. Int J Cancer 26:703–709

Karjalainen S, Hakulinen T (1988) Survival and prognostic factors of patients with skin melanoma. Cancer 62:2274–2280

Lee JAH (1991) Trends in melanoma incidence and mortality. Clin Dermatol (in press)

Lemish WM, Heenan PJ, Holman CDJ, Armstrong BK (1983) Survival from preinvasive and invasive malignant melanoma in Western Australia. Cancer 52:580–585

Lindegard B (1990) Mortality and fatality of cutaneous malignant melanoma in Sweden, 1982–1986. Biomed Pharmacother 44:495–501

Longstreth JD (1987) Ultraviolet radiation and melanoma. With a special focus on assessing the risks of stratospheric ozone depletion. US Environmental Protection Agency, Washington, DC

Muir CS, Nectoux J (1982) Time trends: malignant melanoma of the skin. In: Magnus K (ed.) Trends in cancer incidence. Hemisphere Publishing Corporation, Washington, pp 365–385

Nordlund JJ, Kirkwood J, Forget BM et al. (1985) Demographic study of clinically atypical (dysplastic) nevi in patients with melanoma and comparison subjects. Cancer Res 45:1855–1861

Osterlind A. (1987) Trends in incidence of ocular malignant melanoma in Denmark, 1943–1982 Int J Cancer 40:161–164

Osterlind A (1990) Malignant melanoma in Denmark: occurrence and risk factors. Acta Oncol 29:833–853

Osterlind A, Tucker MA, Stone BJ et al. (1988a) The Danish case-control control study of cutaneous malignant melanoma. II. Importance of UV-light exposure. Int J Cancer 42:319–324

Osterlind A, Hou-Jensen K, Jensen OM (1988b) Incidence of cutaneous malignant melanoma in Denmark, 1978–1982. Atomic site distribution, histologic types, and comparisons with non-melanoma skin cancer. Br J Cancer 58:385–391

Osterlind A, Engholm G, Jensen OM (1988c) Trends in cutaneous malignant melanoma in Denmark, 1943–1982, by anatomic site. APMIS 1988c; 96:953–963

Reilly WK, Administrator, US Environmental Protection Agency (1991) Text of Public Statement: April

Roush GC, Schymura MJ, Holford TR (1985) Risk for cutaneous melanoma in recent Connecticut birth cohorts. Am J Public Health 75:679–682

Schneider JS, Sagebiel RW, Moore II DH, Lawton GM (1987) Melanoma surveillance and earlier diagnosis. Lancet i:1435

Schultz S, Kane M, Roush R et al. (1990) Time to recurrence varies inversely with thickness in clinical stage 1 cutaneous melanoma. Surg Gynecol Obstet 171:393–397

Scotto, J, Cotton G, Urbach F et al. (1987) Biologically effective ultra-violet radiation: surface measurements in the United States, 1974 to 1985. Science 239:762–764

Scotto J, Pitcher H, Lee JAH (1991) Indications of decreasing trends in skin melanoma risks among whites in the United States. Int J Cancer 49:1–7

Strickland D, Lee JAH (1981) Melanomas of the eye: stability of rates. Am J Epidemiol 113:700–702

Thorn M, Adami H-O, Bergstrom R et al. (1989) Trends in survival from malignant melanoma: remarkable improvement in 23 years. J Natl Cancer Inst 81:611–617

van der Esch EP, Muir CS, Nectoux J et al. (1991) Temporal change in diagnostic criteria as a cause of the increase of malignant melanoma over time is unlikely. Int J Cancer 47:183 190

Venzon DJ, Moolgavkar SH (1984) Cohort analysis of malignant melanoma in five countries. Am J Epidemiol 119:62–70

Weinstock MA, Colditz GA, Willett WC et al. (1991) Recall (report) bias and reliability in the retrospective assessment of melanoma risk. Am J Epidemiol 133:240–245

2 Clinical Differential Diagnosis of Cutaneous Malignant Melanoma

Rona M. MacKie

Introduction

The clinical differential diagnosis of malignant melanoma has to be approached at three levels. At the most advanced level, the expert must be aware of a wide range of possibilities and must make a reasoned judgement as to what procedures are necessary to confirm his clinical impression, and thereafter institute appropriate therapy. At the level of general practice, the family doctor him or herself, should be aware of a reasonable range of diagnostic possibilities and be aware of clinical features which can help in assessment. The most obvious example here is that most family doctors should be able to distinguish between seborrhoeic keratoses or basal cell papillomas and melanocytic lesions. The third level is recognition of pigmented lesions which may have serious significance on the part of the patient. At this level it is important not to expect more than can be reasonably required of the general public. It is generally agreed that the most consistent feature of an early malignant melanoma is change. This is sensitive but is not specific, but if the public are advised that any new or changing pigmented lesions in an adult should be shown to their medical adviser, in general, tragedies will be avoided.

At the level of expert clinical differential diagnosis, it must never be forgotten that this is not an absolute art. The role of clinical differential diagnosis is in making a reasoned decision about future pathological confirmation of a clinical impression. Most studies suggest that clinical prehistological accuracy is correct in around 50% of cases if relatively inexperienced practitioners are tested, and that well-trained experts can attain a prebiopsy diagnostic accuracy of around 86%. In a condition with as serious significance as malignant melanoma, there is no place for decisions on management based on other than pathological confirmation.

However, it is also important for the clinician to recognize that the pathological diagnosis of early malignant melanoma is not an absolute art, although there is no doubt that the range of doubtful lesions can be cut down considerably by comparison with the clinical situation. The experienced dermatopathologist will have no trouble whatever in distinguishing early malignant melanoma from non-melanocytic lesions which could clinically cause diagnostic confusion. Examples of such lesions include seborrhoeic keratoses, angiomas and dermatofibromas. However, the borderline area between the so-called dysplastic naevus and early invasive malignant melanoma can be very blurred, and a range of opinions will be obtained if a range of experienced pathologists are consulted. This is becoming increasingly important with the large number of patients now presenting with thin, good prognosis lesions. It is generally in this area of thin lesions that the greatest area of pathological discrepancy lies.

Other areas of possible pathological discrepancy include the differentiation between Spitz naevi and Spitzoid melanomas, and also in the rare, and at times, elusive desmoplastic melanoma. In this chapter, the clinical differential diagnosis of melanoma will be discussed in terms of the clinically and pathologically recognizable histogenetic subsets. The four main groups are lentigo maligna melanoma, superficial spreading melanoma, nodular melanoma, and acral lentiginous melanoma.

The concept of these histogenetically distant subsets was introduced by Clark et al. (1969) and is based on clinical and pathological features. Ackerman (1982) has suggested that these subsets are not pathologically relevant and that all melanoma arises from the one starting point. It is, of course, absolutely accurate that all melanoma begins with a proliferation of neoplastic melanocytes, but the tempo and steps involved thereafter in the progression from a small area of focal neoplastic transformation in situ of the melanocytic system to vertically invasive, potentially metastatic melanoma, are different. Because of this, the clinical differential diagnosis of the different growth patterns varies and they therefore have relevance in the context of this chapter.

Patients at Risk of Developing Melanoma

It is important to consider the clinical differential diagnosis of malignant melanoma in the context of the patient, not just of the pigmented lesion. The great majority of malignant melanomas occur in adults, and in the Scottish Melanoma Group's series of over 4000 melanomas, only 12 prepubertal lesions are registered (MacKie et al. in preparation). Once puberty is reached, the age-specific incidence of melanoma rises steadily with each decade. In the Scottish series the mean age at diagnosis of cutaneous melanoma is 53 years. In the younger males and females the most likely sites for melanoma to develop are the lower leg in women, and on the back in men. In the over-65 age group, melanomas in both sexes are commonest on the face, although only half of these, are of the lentigo maligna melanoma type.

The person at greatest risk of developing melanoma may have a variety of identifiable phenotypic and environmental features. Patients at greatest risk of primary malignant melanoma are, first, those who have already had one primary tumour. Patients who have already had one primary malignant melanoma develop a second quite unrelated primary tumour in around 8% of cases. It is, therefore, important that all patients who have had primary melanoma are well checked at follow-up visits, not just in the scar and nodal draining area, but also have a total body skin examination. Furthermore, these patients should be instructed on the recognition of early malignant melanoma so that they can recognize any change and report this between regular follow-up visits.

The relatively rare group of patients with familial melanoma and also multiple atypical or dysplastic naevi, are also at increased risk of malignant melanoma. The relative risk of malignant melanoma developing varies according to the NIH A, B, C and D classification for dysplastic naevus syndrome (National Institutes of Health 1984). It is important to establish when a patient with new malignant melanoma presents whether or not this patient falls into the category of familial melanoma. Patients are surprisingly ill-informed about the medical history of their relatives, and full examination of first-degree relatives is strongly recommended.

Other recognized risk factors include a childhood spent in a tropical or similar environment, and a history of severe blistering sunburn. The phenotype of the patient at greater than average risk of melanoma, is that of an individual who has large numbers (50 or greater) of banal pigmented melanocytic naevi, who has a freckling tendency, and who has three or more large clinically atypical naevi greater than 3mm in largest diameter. All of these features should help to define around 20% of the population who are likely to develop 50% of cutaneous malignant melanomas. Thus although these features are useful pointers, they are by no means totally specific.

Lentigo Maligna Melanoma

Primary cutaneous lentigo maligna melanoma usually has a very slow phase of preinvasive evolution. This preinvasive phase is termed the lentigo maligna phase and may exist for five to ten years before invasion from the epidermis into the dermis develops. Of all lentigo malignas which proceed to lentigo maligna melanoma 90% develop on the face, with the remaining 10% on other chronically sun-exposed sites, such as the back of the hand or the lower leg. The lentigo maligna patient is also at greater risk of developing non-melanoma skin cancer, including basal and squamous cell carcinoma.

The first signs of the preinvasive lentigo maligna phase is the development, usually on the face, of a slowly expanding, irregular, brown or black, macular lesion (Fig. 2.1). Over a period of a year or two, this may reach a size of 5–10 mm in largest diameter and, as the outer margin extends laterally, there may be some central clearance of pigmentation giving rise to a relatively depigmented and sometimes mildly scarred area. This phenomenon of partial regression, is extremely common in lentigo malignas.

If left untreated and observed, this lentigo maligna may reach a size of several centimetres in largest diameter, with a highly irregular outline and irregular, but still macular, central pigmentation. After an unpredictable period of time, however, a proportion of lentigo malignas progress to the next stage of tumour development with the appearance of a vertically invasive nodule, usually densely black in colour, of invasive malignant melanocytes (Fig. 2.2). This is the point at which the epidermis is breached and dermal invasion is seen on pathological examination. Once an invasive lentigo maligna melanoma has developed, we and others have observed that thickness for thickness these tumours have the same prognosis as lesions of other histogenetic types. The biological difference is that the time taken to reach a Breslow thickness of, for example, 2 mm is very much longer in the slowly evolving lentigo maligna melanoma than in the rapidly evolving nodular melanoma.

The main clinical differential diagnosis of the lentigo maligna melanoma type of lesion is the flat seborrhoeic keratosis. This is illustrated in Fig. 2.3, where it will be seen that this lesion has a rather dull surface with small horn cysts clearly visible on moderate magnification. The extensive lateral irregularity and central clearing of pigment so typical of lentigo maligna melanoma is not seen in seborrhoeic keratosis.

A second lesion which may require to be differentiated from lentigo maligna melanoma is the pigmented actinic keratosis, well shown in Fig. 2.4. This particular lesion usually has a greater degree of inflammation and crusting and a lesser degree of melanin pigmentation than the lentigo maligna melanoma.

If clinical doubt persists on examination of an irregular pigmented lesion on the face of an elderly individual, an incisional biopsy in this situation is usually permissible to identify the cell type involved, the biological nature of the lesion and to make reasonable decisions about further management, including the necessity or otherwise of complete excision of the lesion, or the possibility of non-surgical therapy. Incisional biopsies in general, however, are not normal procedure in suspected melanoma, and this decision should be left to an individual with some experience of dealing with pigmented lesions.

Superficial Spreading Malignant Melanoma

Of all melanomas in the UK 50% are of the superficial spreading type, and this is therefore the lesion which is most likely to be diagnosed or suspected in the family doctor's surgery. The typical site is on the lower leg, and the most likely patient is female, as twice as many women as men in the UK suffer from melanoma (Fig. 2.5). The classical early superficial spreading melanoma currently has a diameter of around 7 mm, and is an irregularly shaped, expanding, brown or black lesion (Fig. 2.6). The lesion is both grossly asymmetrical and also has pronounced small irregularities around the periphery. In addition, there is usually striking variation in brown and black pigmentation within the lesion. These shades of brown and black may be admixed with both red, indicating an inflammatory infiltrate within the lesion, and also blue or white, indicating some degree of partial regression.

An important point with these lesions is, first, that the early melanoma looks distinctly different from the surrounding banal pigmented naevi. Individuals vary in their tendency to develop naevi, and also vary in the size and colour intensity of naevi which develop. Early melanomas, however, look distinctly different from

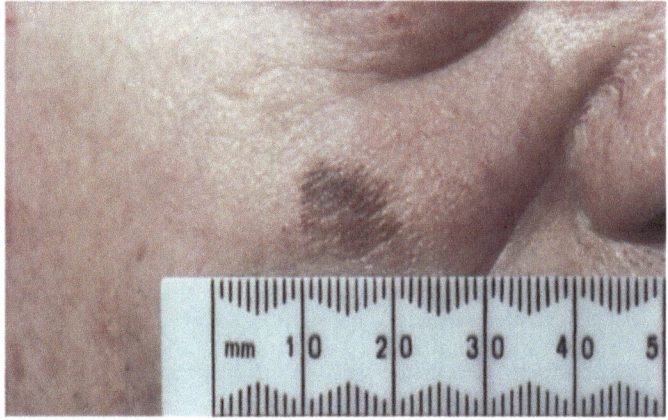

Fig. 2.1. Lentigo maligna, showing flat area of pigmentation on cheek.

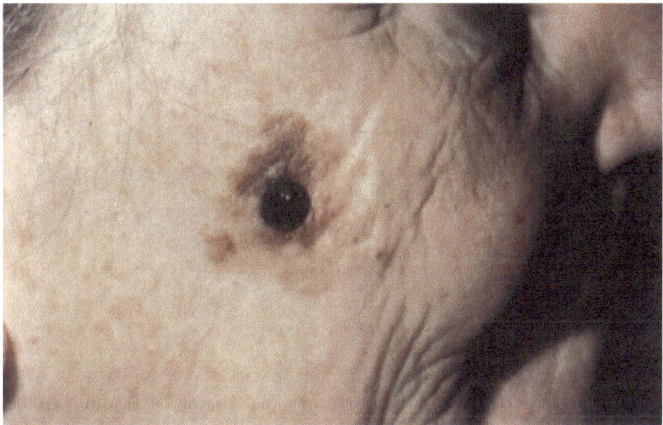

Fig. 2.2. Lentigo maligna melanoma. Note elevated nodule in the centre of flat pigmentation.

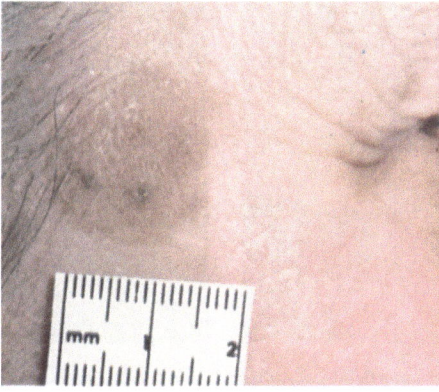

Fig. 2.3. Flat seborrhoeic keratosis on the cheek. Note dull, non-reflective surface.

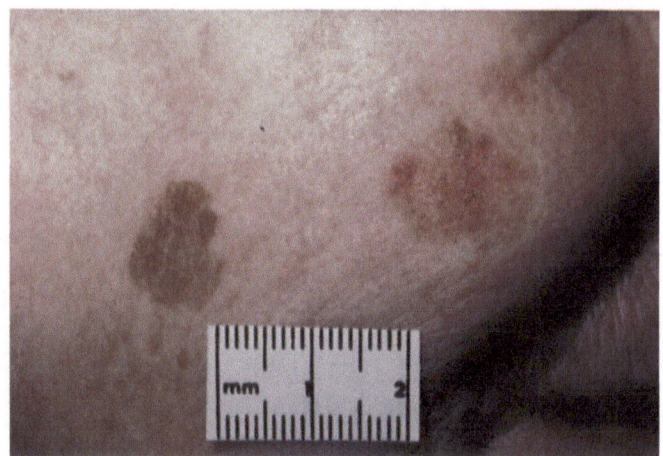

Fig. 2.4. Actinic keratosis to the right and seborrhoeic keratosis to the left illustrate the erythematous element present, usually in actinic keratoses.

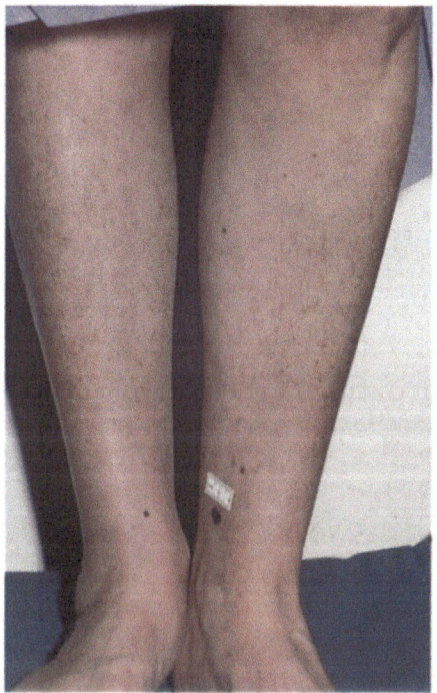

Fig. 2.5. Distant view of superficial spreading melanoma on the anterior aspect of the ankle of a female leg.

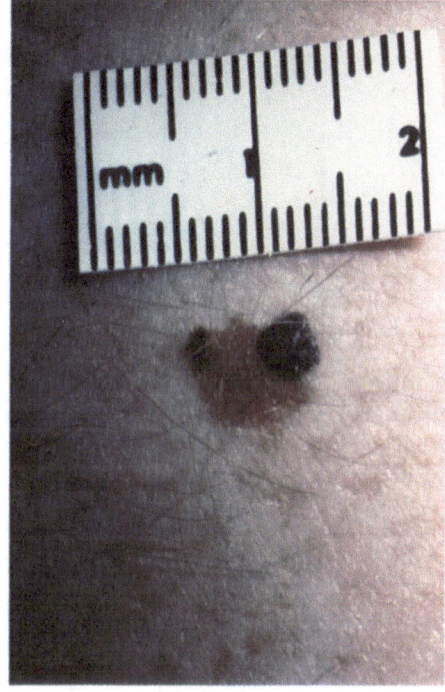

Fig. 2.6. Close-up view of superficial spreading melanoma, showing irregular outline and irregular pigmentation.

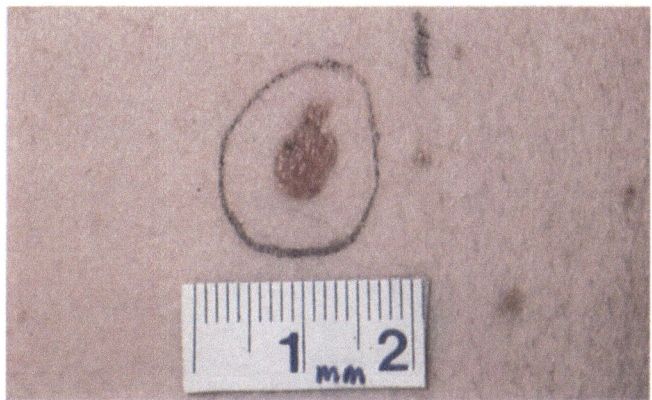

Fig. 2.7. Clinically atypical and pathologically dysplastic naevus showing striking irregularity of outer margin.

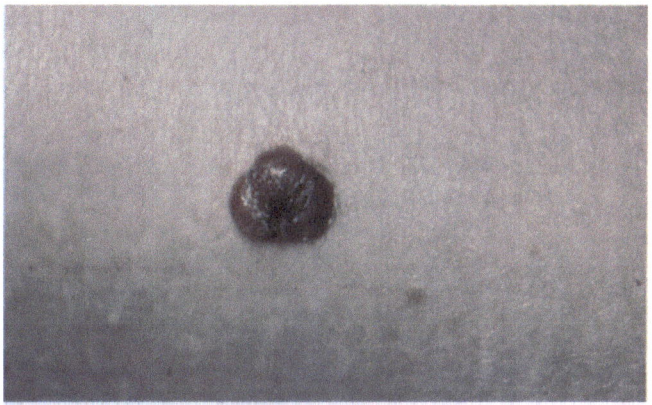

Fig. 2.8. Relatively non-pigmented nodular melanoma.

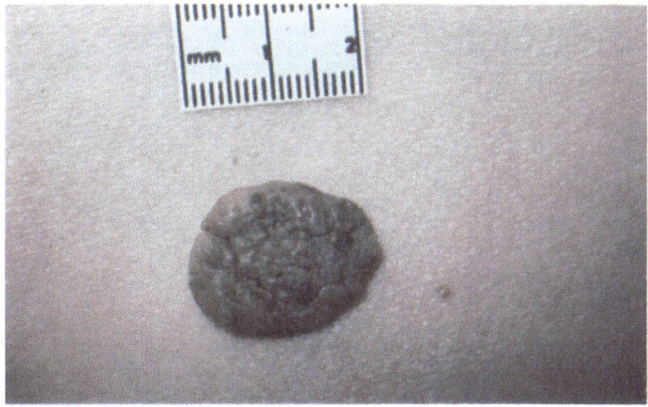

Fig. 2.9. Densely pigmented, elevated seborrhoeic keratosis.

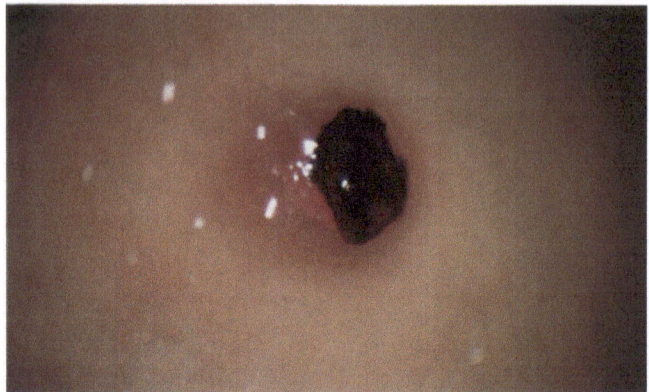

Fig. 2.10. Sclerosed angioma. Note how moderate magnification and covering the surface with oil renders the pigment clearly vascular in origin.

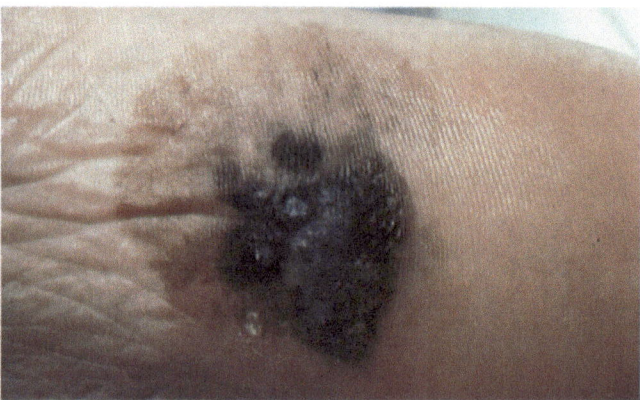

Fig. 2.11. Acral lentiginous melanoma. Note macular component surrounding elevated darker area.

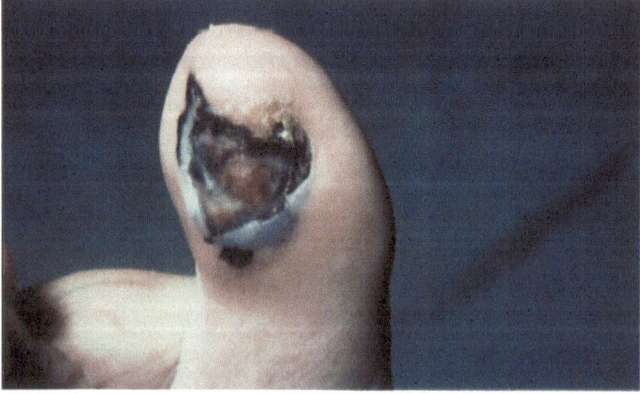

Fig. 2.12. Periungual melanoma on hallux. Note gross loss of normal nail tissue.

the naevi on the anatomical site of the individual. Most patients, with help, are good at recognizing early malignant melanoma, and the feature which they most commonly draw to their medical attendant's attention is the presence of change in either the size, the shape, or the colour of a pigmented lesion. This may be change in size, shape and colour of a pre-existing, presumed benign, melanocytic naevus, or the appearance of a new pigmented lesion in an adult which proceeds to change in size, shape and colour. This history of change should never be ignored, no matter how banal the individual lesion looks on cursory examination.

The seven-point checklist devised in Glasgow on a population of melanomas first seen in 1984, was revised in 1989 following changes in the population presenting to our pigmented lesion clinic with malignant melanoma after a public education campaign. The revised seven-point checklist (Table 2.1) shows that change in size, shape and colour of a new or pre-existing pigmented lesion are all regarded as major signs of early malignant melanoma, particularly of the superficial spreading type. Minor signs are a diameter of 7 mm or greater, the presence of inflammation, the presence of any oozing or sticking of the lesion to overlying clothing, and the presence of mild sensory change. Oozing and crusting as distinct from frank bleeding is seen even in thin melanomas, and a common reason given by women for seeking medical advice about a new or changing pigmented lesion on the leg is that the lesion was sticking to stockings or tights.

Taken together these features are all helpful in identifying early malignant melanoma but are neither totally sensitive nor totally specific. At the present time there is no technique for identifying melanoma prebiopsy that is 100% sensitive and 100% specific, and until this is available, aids to recognition, such as the Glasgow seven-point checklist, or the American A, B, C, Ds, should be regarded as useful guides to identifying lesions for further investigation or possible biopsy rather than absolute rules.

Lesions which may cause clinical confusion with early superficial spreading melanoma are most often benign melanocytic naevi and occasionally atypical seborrhoeic keratoses. The benign melanocytic naevi which most often cause problems include the so-called dysplastic naevi, or clinically atypical naevi and also combined naevi where pathological examination shows a combination of a compound naevus and also a blue naevus.

Clinically atypical naevi have a diameter of greater than 5 mm, and one at least of an irregular outline, irregular colour or inflammation. Fig. 2.7 shows one such

Table 2.1. Clinical features of early malignant melanoma: seven-point checklist

Major features	1. Change in size of previous lesion or obvious growth of new lesion
	2. Irregular shape – asymmetry and an irregular outline of a newly developed pigmented lesion or appearance of this feature in an old lesion
	3. Irregular colour – a variety of shades of brown and black in a new or old lesion
Minor features	4. Largest diameter 7 mm or greater. Most benign acquired naevi are smaller than this
	5. Inflammation – rare in benign lesions unless they are regularly traumatized
	6. Oozing, crusting or bleeding. Oozing, causing sticking of clothing such as stockings to the lesion, is relatively common in early melanoma. It is not seen in naevi.
	7. Change in sensation – usually described as mild itch

lesion. Without pathological confirmation it is virtually impossible to be certain one is not dealing with an early superficial spreading malignant melanoma when faced with such a lesion. Depending on clinical circumstances and the patient's other lesions, many of these lesions may have to be removed for pathological examination. An alternative approach, however, in a major centre with appropriate photographic facilities available, is to record these lesions photographically and then to view the patient at regular intervals, possibly three-monthly, with the photographs to hand. We and others have shown that this is a safe method of identifying extremely early malignant change, and the need for multiple biopsies is thus reduced.

Nodular Melanoma

In the experience of most individuals who see many melanomas, nodular malignant melanoma is the most difficult lesion to diagnose confidently on clinical grounds. Here the history is usually of fairly rapid growth, often over six to eight weeks or a few months, rather than many months or years. The lesion is frequently uniformly round or oval and elevated. Crusting and bleeding are early features of this lesion, even when it has not yet reached a diameter of 1 cm. The colour is often a uniform red, grey or black, and the red lesions are, of course, the amelanotic melanomas which give rise to most clinical confusion (Fig. 2.8). The differential diagnosis here will lie between vascular lesions, either benign or malignant, and also possibly dermatofibromas and deeply pigmented seborrhoeic keratoses (Fig. 2.9). Vascular lesions are generally uniformly red, and examination of the lesion, having first covered it with mineral oil, and using moderate magnification and a bright light, may help to identify the fact that the pigment present is blood clot rather than melanocytic (Fig. 2.10). Dermatofibromas are often rather firm, slower growing lesions than nodular melanomas and the bulk of the lesion will be under the skin surface.

Acral or Acral Lentiginous Melanoma

The acral or acral lentiginous melanoma is usually found on the soles of the feet, and in our Scottish series eight times as many lesions are found on this site as on the hands. The early lesion has a similar lentiginous spreading pattern to that of lentigo maligna, but over a period of months a raised invasive component develops, usually centrally (Fig. 2.11). As with superficial spreading lesions the cardinal features are change, with irregularity of colour and an irregular outer edge.

A subset of acral melanomas are the subungual melanomas. The majority of these are found around the big toe-nail (Fig. 2.12), for reasons which are not understood, and here there is evidence for clinical delay and inappropriate management on the part of both hospital and family doctors. All those involved in identifying early malignant melanoma should beware of pigmentation around the toe-nail, particularly of the big toe, and should immediately arrange for an appropriate diagnostic procedure to be carried out in the case of any pigmented lesion in which there is pigmentation on the skin of the dorsum of the toe adjacent to the actual nail.

The clinical differential diagnosis of acral melanomas on the soles of the feet usually lies between benign naevi and melanoma, although occasionally pigmented plantar warts may confuse the issue. In the case of subungual melanomas, the differential diagnosis may lie between pigmentation due to haemorrhage because of trauma or pigmentation due to the presence of a fungal infection.

Aids to Clinical Diagnosis

The operation microscope and the dermatoscope are both useful in identifying features on the surface of pigmented lesions which may assist in clinical prebiopsy recognition. Examination of the surface of the lesion at a magnification of ×10 having previously applied mineral oil to the skin to clear the surface stratum corneum can enhance diagnostic accuracy. This is particularly true for angiomas as the oil application makes the nature of the pigment clear in the majority of cases. The dermatoscope is a portable and less-expensive development, similar in size to an otoscope. Although potentially useful, no clinical study has yet demonstrated an advance in diagnostic accuracy using this apparatus in comparison with for example a hand lens and good illumination.

In conclusion, it must always be remembered that the clinical differential diagnosis of pigmented lesions with the possibility of early melanoma is a prelude to pathological confirmation. Nowadays the great majority of melanomas are identified when they are small, i.e. less than 1.5 cm in largest diameter. If there is any clinical possibility whatsoever of malignant melanoma, the correct procedure is to arrange for an excision biopsy to be carried out with a narrow margin of surrounding normal skin, and thereafter to obtain pathological confirmation of the diagnosis and to plan appropriate therapy. There is no evidence that this two-stage surgical approach is associated with any deterioration in prognosis.

References

Ackerman AB (1982) Disagreements about classification of malignant melanomas. Am J Dermatopathol 29:705–726

Clark EH, From L, Bernardino EA, Mihm MC (1969) The histiogenesis and biologic behaviour of primary malignant melanomas of the skin. Cancer Res 29:705–726

National Institutes of Health (1984) Consensus Conference. Precursors to malignant melanoma. JAMA 251:1864–1866

MacKie RM, Hole D, Aitchison et al. (1991) Cutaneous melanoma in Scotland 1979–89. (in preparation)

3 Differential Diagnosis of Malignant Melanoma by Algorithm

R. E. Ashton

Malignant melanoma may be confused with other skin lesions. It is important to know what these are, so that they may be considered and excluded in the differential diagnosis. A series of algorithms are presented here to aid in this differential diagnosis.

In order to make any clinical diagnosis in dermatology certain key physical signs must be interpreted correctly so that the most appropriate algorithm is selected. These are:

1. Erythematous or non-erythematous, i.e. if red/pink, does this whiten on pressure?
2. Surface features i.e. is the surface:
   a) not different from surrounding skin (smooth/normal)
   b) crusted, ulcerated or bleeding
   c) warty
3. If the surface is smooth/normal, then also establish:
   a) if it is flat (macule/patch) or raised (papule/nodule/plaque)
   b) the colour (brown, black, red, orange etc.).

Malignant melanoma should be considered in the differential diagnosis of the following:

1. Brown or black lesions which have a smooth/normal surface,
   a) flat lesions (macules/patches) (see Fig. 3.1)
   b) raised lesions (papules/nodules/plaques) (see Figs 3.2 and 3.3)
2. Ulcerated, crusted or bleeding lesions (see Fig. 3.4)
3. Any rapidly growing red/purple lesion (see Figs 3.5 and 3.6)
4. Warty (brown) lesions (included as these often worry patients especially if they have been traumatized and bled) (see Fig. 3.7)

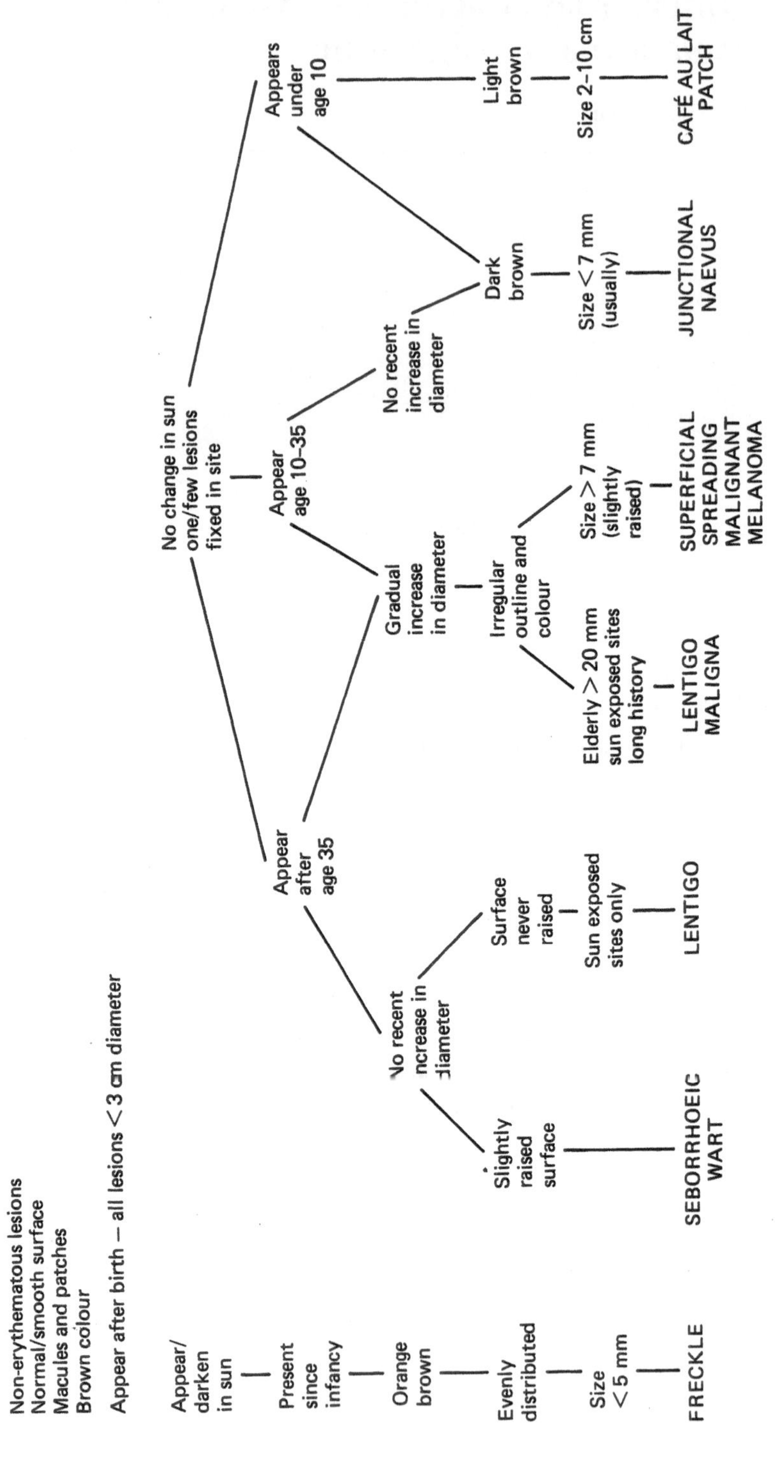

Non-erythematous lesions
Normal/smooth surface
Macules and patches
Brown colour

Appear after birth — all lesions < 3 cm diameter

No change in sun one/few lesions fixed in site

Appear/darken in sun

Appear after age 35

Appear age 10-35

Appears under age 10

No recent increase in diameter

Gradual increase in diameter

No recent increase in diameter

Dark brown

Light brown

Present since infancy

Orange brown

Evenly distributed

Size < 5 mm

FRECKLE

Slightly raised surface

SEBORRHOEIC WART

Surface never raised

Sun exposed sites only

LENTIGO

Irregular outline and colour

Elderly > 20 mm sun exposed sites long history

LENTIGO MALIGNA

Size > 7 mm (slightly raised)

SUPERFICIAL SPREADING MALIGNANT MELANOMA

Size < 7 mm (usually)

JUNCTIONAL NAEVUS

Size 2-10 cm

CAFÉ AU LAIT PATCH

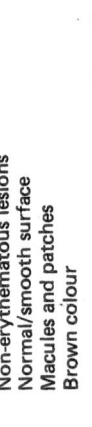

Fig. 3.1.

Freckles (Ephelides)

These are small (1–5 mm in diameter) orangy-brown macules which appear and increase in number and in size with sun exposure. They are commoner in red-haired, blue-eyed individuals who burn rather than tan in the sun. Histologically they contain normal numbers of melanocytes but increased melanin pigment. They do not usually present a diagnostic problem.

Seborrhoeic Warts

When they first arise they may present as flat brown lesions, but after a time become raised. They may be confused with lentigos since both occur in the elderly on sun exposed sites. Close inspection of the surface should show that they are slightly elevated.

Lentigo

Lentigoes are larger and darker than freckles and may have irregular edges. They occur mainly on sun exposed skin but are present all the year round. Their numbers increase with increasing age: they need to be differentiated from a lentigo maligna. Histologically there are increased numbers of melanocytes in the basal layer.

Lentigo Maligna (Hutchinson's Freckle)

This looks very similar to an ordinary lentigo, but is larger (>20 mm), has irregular edges and variation in pigment. It occurs only on sun-damaged skin, most commonly on the cheeks of the elderly. It may be difficult to distinguish from a benign lentigo, but slow extension over several years is characteristic. Histologically it is a malignant melanoma confined to the epidermis (malignant melanoma-in-situ).

Junctional Naevus

A flat (sometimes slightly elevated) dark-brown mole with regular well-defined borders. Most are smaller than 7 mm in diameter. They can occur anywhere on the skin. Histologically groups of melanocytes are found in contact with the basal layer but budding down into the dermis.

Superficial Spreading Malignant Melanoma

The early growth phase of a malignant melanoma is horizontal with migration of the neoplastic cells outwards along the dermoepidermal junction. This change is seen clinically as a junctional naevus enlarging in diameter, with variation in degree of pigmentation and an irregular border often with scalloped edges (see also nodular melanoma).

Café au Lait Patch

These are light-brown macules, round or oval in shape, and often large (2–10 cm diameter). They are present at birth or appear in early childhood. If more than six are found, or if present in the axilla, a diagnosis of neurofibromatosis (von Recklinghausen's disease) is likely. Look also for freckles in the axillae, multiple neurofibromas in the skin or peripheral nerves.

Plane Warts

These are small flat-topped papules but unlike the papules of lichen planus are not shiny. They are not rough to the touch like common warts, but are skin coloured, pink or brown in colour, and may be found in straight lines at sites of trauma (Koebner phenomenon). They occur mainly in children on the dorsum of the hand and on the face.

Skin Tags

Skin tags are small, pedunculated, skin-coloured or brown papules around the neck, in the axillae and sometimes on the upper thighs and eyelids.

Dermatofibroma (Histiocytoma)

This is a firm-hard papule situated in the dermis and occurs anywhere on the body. It is often due to trauma or an insect bite, so is commonly found on ladies'

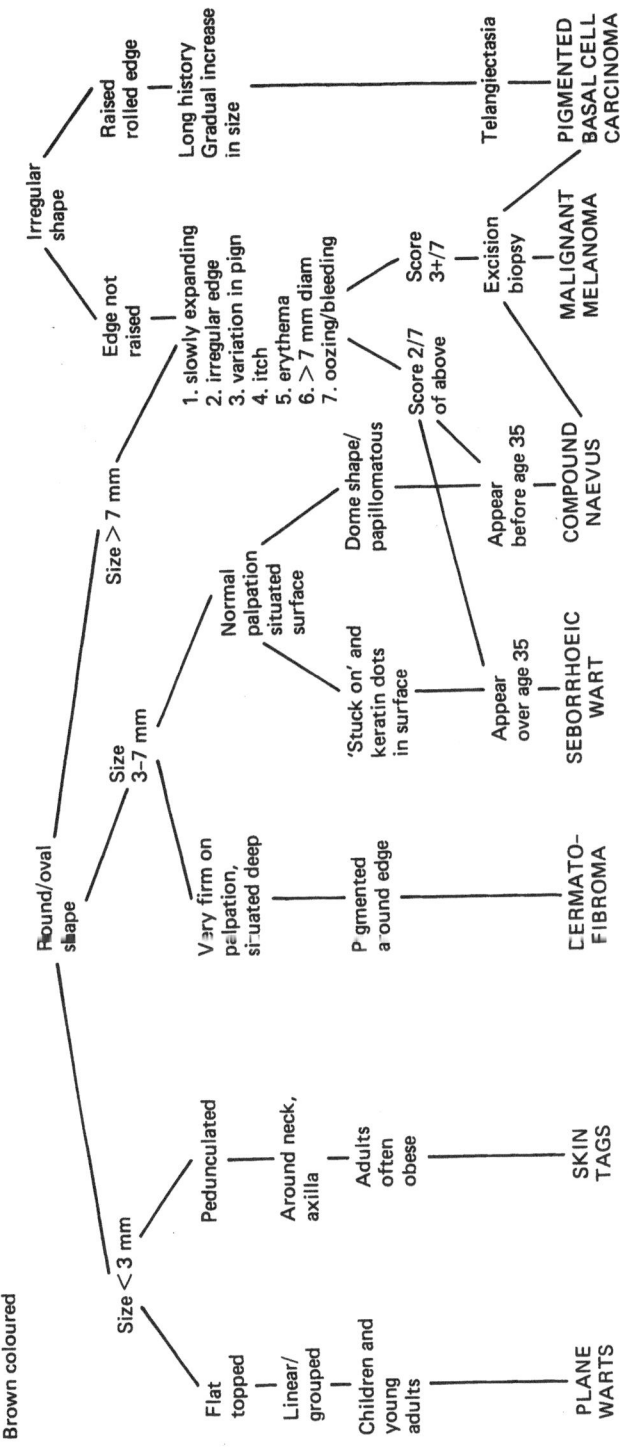

Non-erythematous lesions
Surface normal
Papules, plaques and nodules
Brown coloured

Round/oval shape

Size < 3 mm

Pedunculated

Around neck, axilla

Adults often obese

SKIN TAGS

Flat topped

Linear/ grouped

Children and young adults

PLANE WARTS

Size 3–7 mm

Very firm on palpation, situated deep

Pigmented around edge

DERMATO-FIBROMA

Size > 7 mm

Normal palpation situated surface

Dome shape/ papillomatous

'Stuck on' and keratin dots in surface

Appear over age 35

SEBORRHOEIC WART

Appear before age 35

COMPOUND NAEVUS

1. slowly expanding
2. irregular edge
3. variation in pign
4. itch
5. erythema
6. > 7 mm diam
7. oozing/bleeding

Score 2/7 of above

Score 3+7

Excision biopsy

MALIGNANT MELANOMA

Edge not raised

Irregular shape

Raised rolled edge

Long history
Gradual increase in size

Telangiectasia

PIGMENTED BASAL CELL CARCINOMA

Fig. 3.2.

legs. It is often small ($<5\,mm$), attached to the skin and mobile over deeper structures. The colour can range from skin coloured to pink in the centre and there may be a brown circumference. The surface may be smooth or slightly scaly. Once developed dermatofibromas remain static in size.

Provided the lesion has been palpated, the diagnosis is easy since few common lesions are as hard. Melanocytic naevi are much softer.

Seborrhoeic Wart (Basal Cell Papilloma)

These very common lesions have a flat but warty surface, and typically look as if they are "stuck on" to the skin. Sometimes small keratin cysts can be seen in the surface. Initially they are skin coloured and not very noticeable, but gradually become more prominent and deepen in pigment so that their colour varies through light brown to sometimes jet black. They are often multiple but tend to be isolated rather than in a circumscribed group. With increasing age they occur more frequently and increase in number.

Once the diagnosis has been considered, they should not cause any diagnostic confusion. Their appearance late in life, changing colour, increase in elevation are all features that cause alarm to the patient and result in referral for specialist opinion. Occasionally they may become inflamed, particularly if they have been caught in clothing and partly torn off. They need to be distinguished from moles, solar keratoses, and occasionally from pigmented basal cell carcinoma and malignant melanoma. Moles (melanocytic naevi) are more dome shaped and do not have the "stuck on" appearance, whereas solar keratoses are rough to palpation, being felt more easily than seen. Basal cell carcinoma has a more shiny surface and a rounded edge with telangiectasia, whereas a malignant melanoma shows an irregular edge, colour variation and not the stuck on appearance.

Compound Naevus

These are melanocytic naevi that are both raised and pigmented. Most moles found on the body mature from flat pigmented junctional naevi to raised skin-coloured intradermal naevi. Junctional naevi contain groups (nests) of melanocytes at the dermo-epidermal junction. Gradually the melanocytes drop into the dermis (see Fig. 3.1). This change results in the lesion becoming raised and less pigmented, i.e. a compound naevus, which therefore contains melanocytes both at the dermoepidermal junction (i.e. pigmented) and within the dermis (i.e. raised). Clinically compound naevi vary from a smooth spherical brown papule, to a warty soft brown lesion. It should be recognized that this progression in a mole is a normal benign change and not a sign of malignant change. In fact once the melanocytes drop into the dermis they lose any potential for malignant change.

Non-erythematous lesions
Surface normal
Papules, plaques and nodules
Black/blue colour

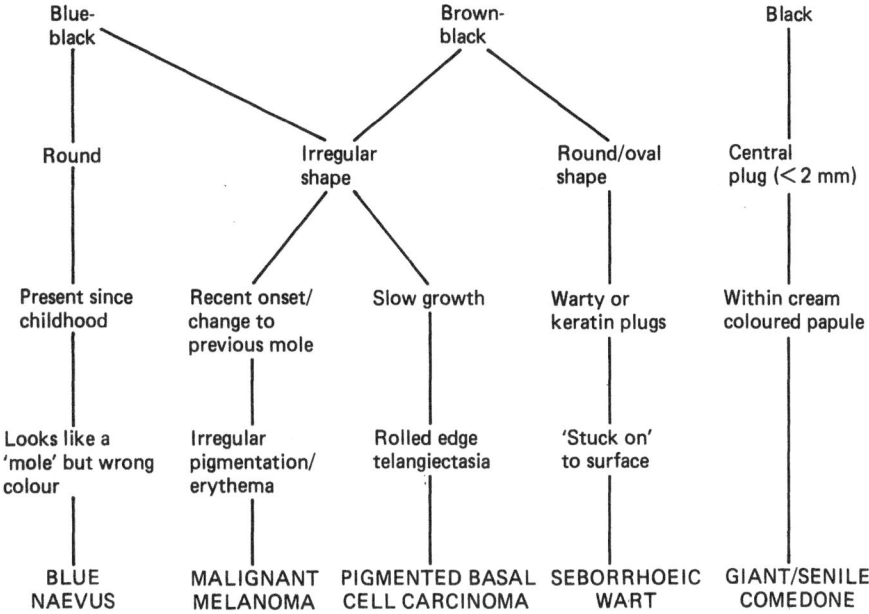

Fig. 3.3.

Nodular Malignant Melanoma

A malignant melanoma is a malignant tumour of melanocytes. Half of these arise from a pre-existing mole which has junctional activity (i.e. a junctional or compound naevus); the other half arise out of normal skin. The initial phase of growth of the melanoma is horizontal along the junction of epidermis and dermis, and is manifest clinically as a superficial spreading melanoma. This type of lesion is flat or only slightly raised. Later (months–years) vertical growth occurs with the melanoma cells invading deeper into the dermis, coming into contact with blood vessels and lymphatics so that metastatic spread is more likely. Clinically the lesion becomes more raised, and the surface may break down with exudation, crusting or bleeding.

There is a direct correlation between the thickness of a melanoma (Breslow thickness – from the top of the granular layer to the deepest point of invasion) and prognosis as measured by survival rates. It is therefore important that malignant melanomas should be diagnosed and removed as early as possible when they are in the horizontal growth phase.

To help in the diagnosis of malignant versus benign moles, a seven-point check list has been devised (Table 3.1). If two or less of the features described are present then one can be confident that a mole is benign. If three or more features

Table 3.1. Checklist of clinical features found in melanomas 2/7 benign; 3 or more for biopsy (courtesy Professor R.M. MacKie, Glasgow University)

1. *Itch*. Benign moles do not itch, malignant melanomas may
2. *Size > 7 mm*. Most malignant lesions have reached 7 mm in diameter before they are recognized, whereas benign lesions are usually smaller.
3. *Increasing size*. Malignant lesions increase in diameter, whereas benign lesions may become more elevated but should never increase in diameter.
4. *Irregular outline*. Benign lesions have a round or oval shape, whereas malignant lesions have a scalloped or notched border.
5. *Colour variation*. Malignant lesions usually show variation in colour from black to light brown, and may even have a reddish tint due to inflammation.
6. *Inflammation*. Benign lesions should never have any evidence of erythema within or around the margin of the lesion.
7. *Crusting/oozing/bleeding*. Can occur in a malignant lesion and may be the reason why the patient has consulted the doctor.

are present then an urgent referral to a dermatologist, or excision of the whole lesion with histological examination is necessary.

Pigmented Basal Cell Carcinoma

Occasionally basal cell carcinomas are heavily pigmented and can be confused with a nodular malignant melanoma, but the typical rolled edge should suggest the correct diagnosis.

Blue Naevus

These look like moles except that they have a dark blue or black colour. They are slightly raised and are usually less than 10 mm diameter. They appear during childhood and then remain fixed, a feature which will distinguish them from a malignant melanoma.

Giant Comedone

Single large comedones can occur on the trunk or face. They are much larger than the blackheads associated with acne but the aetiology is the same. Clinically it is a white/cream papule with a central black punctum. It is unlikely to be confused with a melanoma!

Solar Keratoses

These are typically rough lesions resulting from the production of abnormal keratin in chronically sun-exposed skin. They are commonest on the bald scalp, face and dorsum of the hands, in patients over the age of 50 with fair skin and other evidence of sun damage. Generally they are more easily felt than seen due to the roughness of the abnormal keratin. The surrounding skin may be normal or pink/red. Sometimes scaling is not present and the lesion exists as a fixed pink or brown macule.

The diagnosis should not be difficult as nothing else produces such rough scaling on sun-exposed skin in elderly patients. Seborrhoeic warts occur in similar patients, but never have the same rough feel to palpation, and are generally seen more easily than felt.

Bowen's Disease

This is an intraepidermal squamous cell carcinoma. It looks just like a plaque of psoriasis or eczema, but gradually expands in size over many years and does not respond to topical steroids. The lower leg is the commonest site, but it can be found anywhere on the skin surface.

If multiple lesions are present, particularly if they are not on sun exposed sites, arsenic rather than ultraviolet light may be the cause. Previous arsenic ingestion is confirmed by the presence of rough warty papules on the palms and soles (arsenical keratoses).

Squamous Cell Carcinoma

This is a less common neoplasm of the skin. The older the patient, the more likely the tumour is to be a squamous cell carcinoma. It may arise from a pre-existing lesion such as a solar keratosis or Bowen's disease. Squamous cell carcinomas occur at sites of maximum sun exposure: on a bald head, the lower lip, cheeks, nose, top of ear lobes and dorsum of hands. There is usually other evidence of sun damage such as solar elastosis and solar keratoses. If well differentiated the tumour may initially be scaly or horny; it is differentiated from a solar keratosis by the induration at its base. Later the tumour may ulcerate and then be covered by a crust. The edge of the ulcer is craggy and indurated, whereas the base bleeds easily. It is distinguished from a basal cell carcinoma by its site, the production of keratin and its faster growth (it may grow to 1–2 cm in diameter over a few months). Generally speaking squamous cell carcinomas that arise in sun-damaged skin are less likely to metastasize than squamous cell lesions originating in other parts of the body, e.g. lung.

Squamous cell carcinomas arising in non-sun-exposed skin are usually due to

Non-erythematous/erythematous lesions
Crusted, ulcerated or bleeding surface
Papules, plaques and nodules

Single/few (1–4) lesions, fixed site

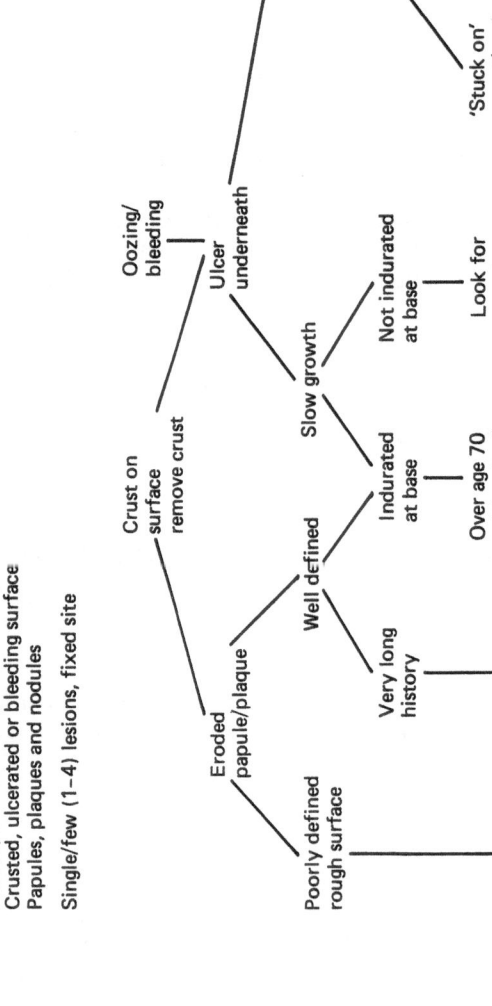

Fig. 3.4.

arsenic, previous radiation, or chronic scars such as in old burn scars, lupus vulgaris or leg ulcers.

Basal Cell Carcinoma (Rodent Ulcer)

This is the commonest malignant tumour of the skin. It usually occurs on exposed areas in people who have had a lot of sun-exposure in the past, and is most common in those with red hair, blue eyes and freckles. Although due to ultraviolet light, it does not occur at sites of maximum sun exposure, i.e. it rarely occurs on the bald scalp, ears, lower lips or backs of hands; sites where squamous cell carcinomas are more common.

A basal cell carcinoma starts as a small papule, pink or pearly in colour usually with obvious telangiectasia over the surface. This gradually enlarges to a nodule or by circumferential growth to produce a flatter lesion (it may only reach a diameter of 1cm over 5 years). It is important to look carefully at the border which tends to be rolled and raised above the centre, like a piece of string around the edge. It may be necessary to stretch the skin to observe this in a very flat lesion. The centre often breaks down forming an ulcer, which may be covered with a serous or blood-stained crust.

Irritated Seborrhoeic Wart

A seborrhoeic wart may be caught in clothing, half torn off and become red and inflamed. It may then be easily mistaken for a mole that has undergone malignant change and result in the patient consulting the doctor. The lesion usually has the "stuck on" appearance of the original lesion, but will have surrounding erythema rather than pigmentation. If the diagnosis is in doubt, it should be removed for histological examination.

Pyogenic Granuloma

This is due to localized overgrowth of blood vessels in response to trauma, often a graze or prick. There is very rapid growth over a few weeks, and usually a history of the lesion having bled spontaneously at some stage. The lesion will be round in shape, bright red or purple in colour, and the surrounding skin will be quite normal. An amelanotic malignant melanoma usually is irregular in shape, has some surrounding pigmentation and grows over a period of months rather than days or weeks.

Non-erythematous lesions
Surface normal
Red/purple/orange colour
Papules, plaques and nodules

No recent increase in size

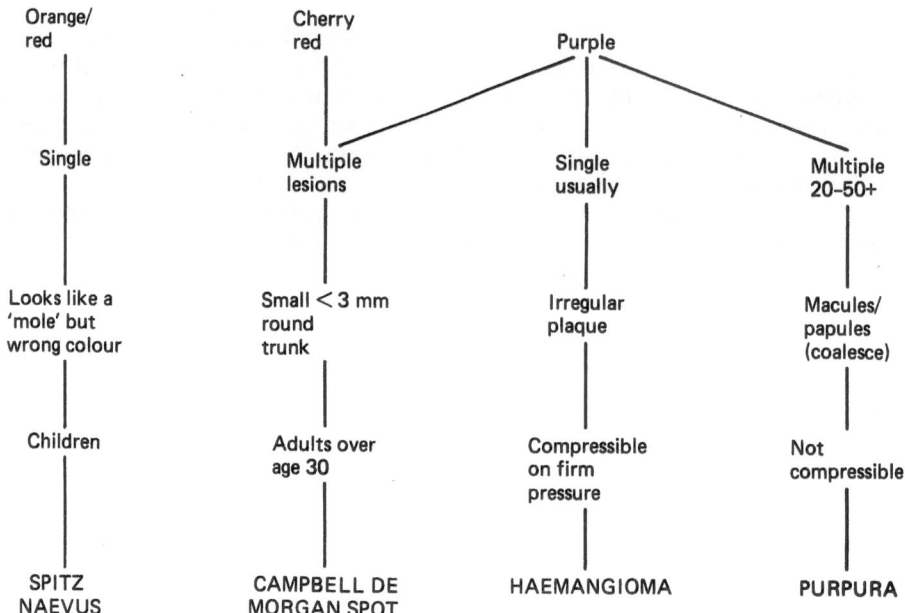

Fig. 3.5.

Spitz Naevus

These look like moles but they are red/orange in colour. In children they cannot be mistaken for anything else. They are not common in adults and if they are removed the histology is found to be very similar to a malignant melanoma, sometimes causing some anxiety: they are, however, benign.

Campbell de Morgan Spot (Cherry Angioma)

These small (1–4 mm) bright red or purple papules appear on the trunk and proximal limbs over the age of 35. They are harmless.

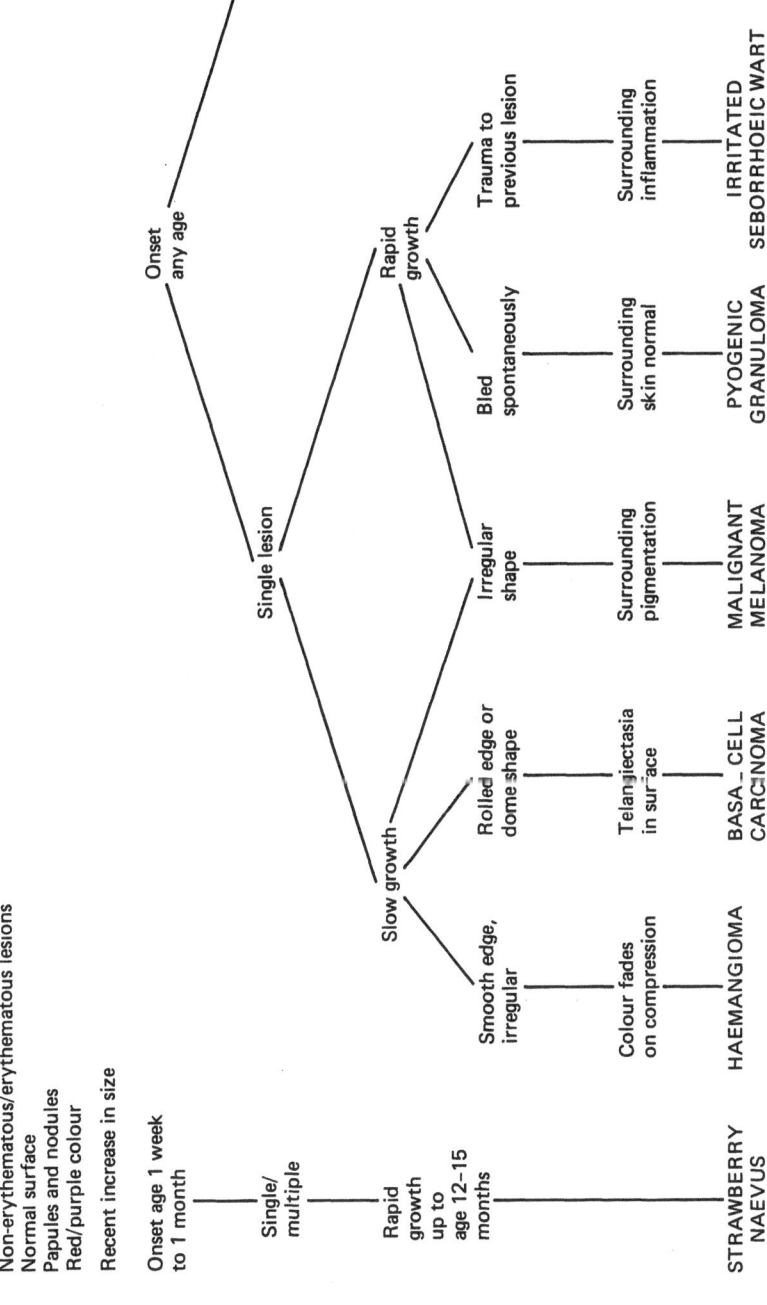

Non-erythematous/erythematous lesions
Normal surface
Papules and nodules
Red/purple colour
Recent increase in size

Onset age 1 week to 1 month

Onset any age

Multiple lesions — All rapid growth — Initially macule becomes papule/nodule — KAPOSI'S SARCOMA

Single lesion

Rapid growth

Trauma to previous lesion — Surrounding inflammation — IRRITATED SEBORRHOEIC WART

Bled spontaneously — Surrounding skin normal — PYOGENIC GRANULOMA

Slow growth

Irregular shape — Surrounding pigmentation — MALIGNANT MELANOMA

Rolled edge or dome shape — Telangiectasia in surface — BASAL CELL CARCINOMA

Smooth edge, irregular — Colour fades on compression — HAEMANGIOMA

Single/multiple — Rapid growth up to age 12–15 months — STRAWBERRY NAEVUS

Fig. 3.6.

Non-erythematous lesions
Warty (papillomatous) surface
Papules, plaques and nodules
Brown/skin colour

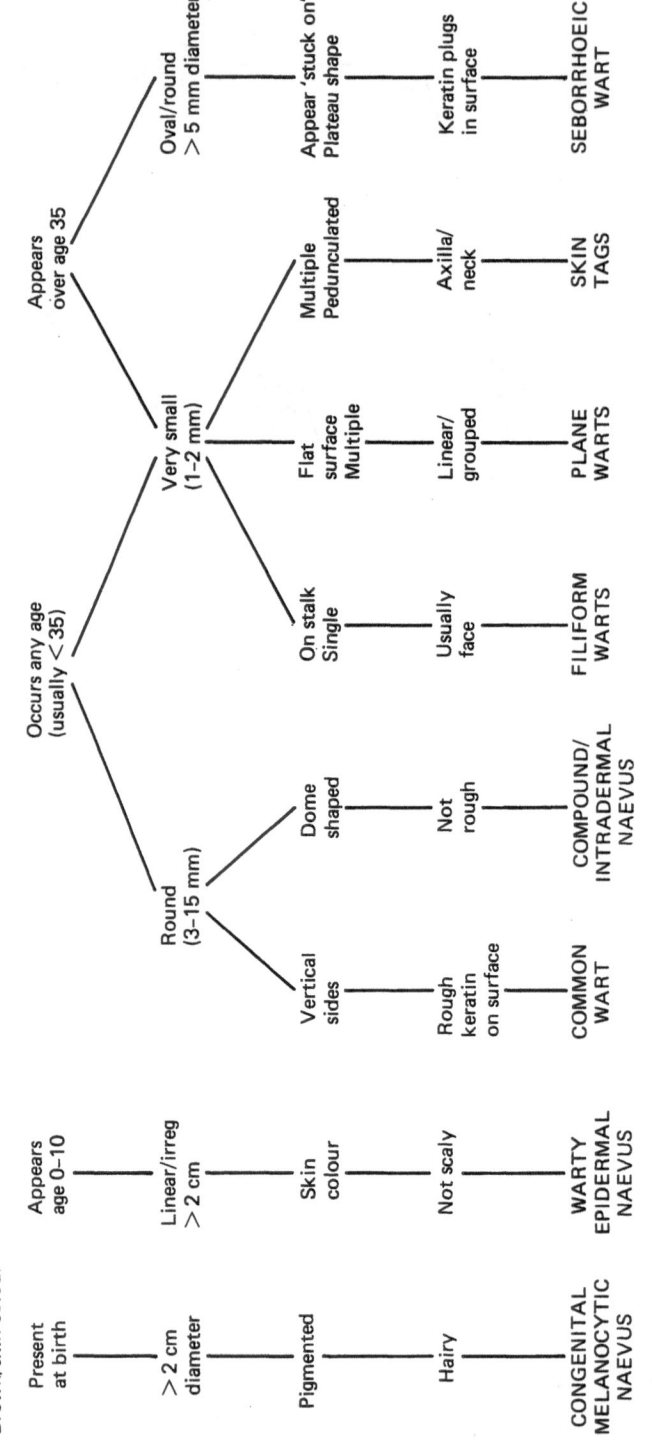

Fig. 3.7.

Haemangioma

Purple papules and plaques which have been present since childhood are due to a localized overgrowth of blood vessel tissue. The stagnant blood within the lesion may be compressed partially, but the colour will never fade completely. Haemangiomas may vary in size, and may occur at any time during childhood.

Acknowledgements.   Sections of this text have been extracted from Ashton RE and Leppard BJ (1990) Differential diagnosis in dermatology. Radcliffe Medical Press, Oxford with permission from the publishers.

4   Clinical Diagnosis of Melanoma

P. Hall

Introduction

For over 150 years it has been realized that the only useful treatment for melanoma is surgery. The single significant advance since then has been the recognition that prompt surgical excision of thin lesions can result in a complete cure. All efforts should be directed towards the detection of these thin lesions. The public must be taught to reveal their changing moles to well-informed family doctors without feeling that they might be wasting their time. These doctors should have a degree of confidence in their ability to diagnose pigmented lesions and have efficient lines of communication to hospital clinicians with a special interest in the disease. The incidence of melanoma in the UK is rising but it is still unlikely that any family doctor will see more than one melanoma in 10 years. Therefore, we cannot expect family doctors to know for certain whether a particular lesion is a melanoma or not, but they must know what might be a melanoma. This chapter summarizes the way in which the different histogenic types of melanoma present, the difficulties that even experienced clinicians have in diagnosis and the tools that have been used to try and help distinguish melanoma from non-melanoma pigmented lesions.

The Patient's History

Normal Moles

Histological features of normal naevi have been found in association with 20%–60% of melanomas and pre-existing moles have been reported by up to 80% of patients with melanoma (Cameron 1968; Sagebiel 1979). It follows, therefore, that the report of a new mole, or a change in a pre-existing mole by a patient requires careful consideration, but not necessarily referral. The majority of us acquire new moles through childhood into early adult life. These lesions will grow in diameter and height, become darker or lighter and may even regress and disappear by the time we are in our forties (Fitzsimmons 1984). Any new mole arising in the late twenties and early thirties and any mole growing out of step compared with other pre-existing naevi at any age including childhood should arouse suspicion. Sudden new growth in a previously dormant mole clearly must be regarded as abnormal. Disorder in growth, border or pattern of pigmentation are the things to watch for (Sober 1985).

Premalignant Lesions

Change in any lesion known to have premalignant potential should make alarm bells ring. Other chapters on aetiology, differential diagnosis and dysplastic naevi will expand the following points.

Congenital Naevi

About 1% of Caucasians are born with naevi (Walton et al. 1976) which can be quite large and sometimes have a warty looking surface. There is a small but unquantified risk of malignant change in these lesions so any change in growth disproportionate to the rate of body growth warrants referral. Whether these lesions should be prophylactically excised is a matter for debate. One certainly could not remove them all for logistical reasons but can, perhaps justify removing those in regions difficult to observe, provided that the wound can be directly closed.

Dysplastic Naevi

A history of more than one family member with a melanoma may suggest that the patient belongs to a small group of families with the dysplastic naevus syndrome and, as such, is at increased risk of melanoma developing either de novo or in one of his naevi. Since up to 8% of the population are reported to have moles satisfying the clinical criteria for dysplastic naevi their presence should be regarded as a marker for increased vigilance rather than a bad omen. These patients especially should be taught to watch for changes in their "funny looking moles" and to avoid unnecessary ultraviolet exposure.

Types of Malignant Melanoma and Presenting Features

Melanomas have been divided into groups according to their patterns of growth. The biological behaviour and therefore the prognosis in each group appear to be different (Clark et al. 1969).

Lentigo Maligna Melanoma

This type accounts for approximately 10%–20% of all melanomas and is a slowly evolving, initially tan-coloured, flat lesion on sun-damaged skin, mainly the face, of persons in their seventies. It increases in size and may undergo many changes in colour with the appearance of dark brown or black areas and in some places the regression of pigmentation leaves blue–grey or even white patches. Often there is a fine reticular pattern of black lines and the border can be very irregular and spidery. This type spends many months or even years growing centrifugally in the epidermis in an "in-situ" radial growth phase. At this stage the terms Lentigo Maligna and Hutchinson's Melanotic Freckle, or Hutchinson's Lentigo, have been used. Once a region of thickening can be detected, progression to an invasive vertical growth phase is likely to have occurred with the attendant capacity for metastasis. Where there is a likelihood that the patient will live long enough for his lesion to develop an invasive component, prophylactic excision, even with skin grafting, is generally advocated. In older and more frail individuals, close follow-up with regular examination and photography to detect early change is a sensible option.

In-Situ Melanoma

As knowledge of the evolution of malignant melanoma in the skin begins to unfold a new variety confined solely to the epidermis has been described (Ackerman 1985). This type is unlikely to be detected before reaching 3–6 mm in diameter as a flat poorly circumscribed asymmetrical lesion with notched, scalloped or jagged borders and mottled brown pigmentation which can be tinged with blue, black or pink. Unlike the lentigo maligna melanoma, these can occur on any part of the body in the younger age groups. Recognition and excision of these preinvasive lesions is now possible with the prospect of complete cure (Todd et al. 1991).

Superficial Spreading Melanoma

In the UK over 50% of melanomas are of this type and affect primarily people in their forties and fifties. Anatomically they are more common on the lower limbs of women and the trunks of men. The female to male preponderance of this lesion is 2:1. The outline is irregular and may be notched and the pigmentation becomes haphazard with hues of tan brown and black. It is not uncommon for pink or white patches to occur where there is tumour regression. The lesion is usually just palpable in the early stages of radial growth but may develop a nodular component as vertical invasion proceeds. Thin, curable lesions will not have the distortion of skin creases and loss of hairs reported in past descriptions since these features will occur only when there is significant tumour activity within the dermis.

Nodular Melanoma

About 25% of melanomas are of this type which affects the middle ages and is more common in men. these melanomas strictly speaking have no radial growth phase and begin immediately to invade vertically. They are the most difficult to diagnose early perhaps because the classical teaching is that these are spherical or "blue-berry" like nodules with a relatively smooth surface and a relatively uniform blue–black colour. It should be possible to detect these melanomas before they reach the dimensions that justify them being termed "Nodular" (a nodule is a circumscribed palpable mass larger than 1 cm in diameter) and before ominous signs of bleeding and ulceration occur. Higgins and du Vivier (1991) regard these signs as dangerously outdated, since lesions detected at this stage are thick and carry a poor prognosis. Their challenge for the 1990s is for these small, darkly growing, melanomas to be detected when their diameters are still around 0.5 cm or less. Thus they have coined the term "papular melanoma" to describe these earlier and more curable lesions (Higgins and du Vivier 1991). At first glance they appear rather regular but close examination of the border frequently reveals an area of notching or a streak of pigment appearing at one edge. The sudden appearance and rapid growth is a major clue in these lesions. Sometimes they appear almost completely depigmented but even in these "Amelanotic melanomas" a rim of pigment is usually left, thereby distinguishing them from the more rapidly growing pyogenic granuloma.

Acral Lentiginous Melanoma

The acral regions are palmar, plantar and subungual areas of the body. It has been debated as to whether all melanomas arising at these sites are from a distinct histopathological category or simply a mixture including some superficial spreading and some nodular type melanomas (Sondergaard 1985). Regardless of these arguments, melanomas arising here seem to have a more aggressive biological behaviour than any of the other types. They can have any of the features described for the types above but unfortunately they tend to be diagnosed when they are much larger and thicker. They are the commonest type of melanoma in Blacks and Oriental people. They are the least common melanoma (approx. 5%) in this country but one which we should feel most pleased about detecting early. A common catch is to treat a dark area on the sole of the foot as a plantar wart, so careful thought about the history and examination findings, including precise location, is needed.

Only 1%–2% of melanomas are in a subungual position and appear as a brown to black discolouration under the nail-bed which may spread onto the nail fold (Hutchinson's sign). The nail plate may become distorted and separate from the nail bed (Shuckla and Hughes 1989). Careful history and examination usually enables these to be distinguished from traumatic haematomas and fungal infections but, where there is doubt, referral for an opinion and careful biopsy must take place and prolonged periods of trial therapy should be avoided.

Screening

Melanoma is an ideal candidate for screening. The prevalence continues to increase, early treatment appears to affect mortality and the screening test is simple and inexpensive. In this country screening is initiated by family doctors whereas in the United States a number of strategies, including "Health Fairs", are employed, with varying results (Koh et al. 1989).

The need for a public education campaign to increase earlier self-recognition of malignant melanoma was highlighted in the UK by Doherty and MacKie (1986) following which seven centres funded by the Cancer Research Campaign were set up in the UK to assess such campaigns during 1986 and 1987. Information was given to general practitioners and the public via leaflets, posters, newspapers, radio and television. The "seven point checklist" (Table 4.1) was adopted by the CRC and formed the basis of an extremely useful booklet for family doctors (MacKie 1985).

A lesion with three or more of the features in the checklist was regarded as suspicious and four features highly likely to be a melanoma.

The results of these campaigns appeared to show an overall increase in the numbers of thin, good-prognosis, tumours diagnosed yet the absolute number of thick lesions remained unchanged (Doherty and MacKie 1988; Whitehead and Wroughton 1988; Graham-Brown et al. 1990). At King's College Hospital London there did appear to be a decrease in absolute numbers of thick melanomas but it was noted that there was a general trend towards thinner lesions presenting over the previous 17 years. This mirrors the apparent worldwide decline in tumour thickness and may signal a change in tumour biology thus making the interpretation of the value of education campaigns difficult (Williams et al. 1990).

It would be unreasonable to expect an aide-memoire such as the seven-point check list to be specific at diagnosing melanomas but one would insist that it be sufficiently sensitive so as never to miss a melanoma. A number of authors have attempted to validate the seven-point checklist and have found areas of deficiency (Keefe et al. 1990a; du Vivier et al. 1990; Higgins et al. 1991). One of these studies (du Vivier et al. 1990) was particularly critical of the choice of 1 cm or more being the important determinant of size since only 50 out of 100 melanomas in their series were as large as this. The ABCDE system of the American Cancer Society: Asymmetry, Border, Colour, Diameter and Elevation is very similar to the seven-point checklist. Both systems suffer from being too orientated towards detecting superficial spreading melanomas which can be thought of as relatively slow-growing lesions waiting to be

Table 4.1.   Original seven-point checklist

---

1. Minor itch or other change in sensation
2. A lesion greater than 1 cm in largest diameter
3. A history of growth or other change in a pigmented lesion in an adult
4. An irregular outline
5. Irregular and varied colours
6. Inflammation in or at the edge of the lesion
7. Bleeding or crusting

Table 4.2.   Revised checklist for suspected malignant melanoma

Major signs	Minor signs
Change in size	Inflammation
Change in shape	Crusting or bleeding
Change in colour	Sensory change
	Diameter 7 mm or more

harvested from the population, while the more biologically aggressive nodular melanomas slip through the net. It is at these nodular melanomas that future education campaigns should be targeted (Keefe et al. 1990b).

Perhaps as a result of these criticisms and from a review of 100 consecutive cases analysed in Glasgow in 1989 the checklist has been revised (MacKie 1989) (Table 4.2). The symptom of itch has been given less emphasis and three major criteria have been isolated such that presence of any one of these warrants referral. Any of the four minor criteria should heighten suspicion but it has been emphasized that the revised checklist must still be thought of as just a guide (MacKie 1990).

The emphasis on change in size, shape, or colour of the lesion makes the checklist more memorable and useful. However, change can be part of the normal life-cycle of a mole (Sober 1985) and some melanomas can be detected when as little as 5 mm in diameter (du Vivier and Higgins 1991). In a recent survey it was found that 19% of melanomas presenting to a pigmented lesion clinic were incidental findings by friends, relatives or doctors (du Vivier et al. 1990) rather than self-referrals. Any new campaigns must target this mode of referral.

Accuracy in Diagnosis

In the UK approximately 20 benign lesions are referred to pigmented lesion clinics by family doctors for every melanoma. This is regarded as an entirely acceptable ratio and suggests that family doctors are very efficiently screening the majority of pigmented lesions. It remains to be seen how the new incentives for General Practitioners to perform minor procedures will affect the referral pattern, most specialists would rather advise about correct management of a lesion than pick up the pieces of an inadequately treated skin malignancy. Furthermore, accurate microstaging particularly of melanoma has such important prognostic information that adequate excision biopsy material must be sent to those who are used to dealing with it.

The clinical diagnosis of melanoma is not always easy even for those professing to have a special interest in the disease. In the 1950s, studies showed that many melanomas were regarded as benign naevi or basal cell papillomas and vice versa (Swerdlow 1952; Becker 1954; McMullan and Hubener 1956). Over the years specialist centres have been publishing data to show how much better they are now compared with before and ratios such as "Diagnostic Accuracy" or "Index of

Suspicion" have been quoted to describe their progress. In the final analysis an impressive sounding index of suspicion in a large American series of 116.7% is attached to a study that still failed to make the correct diagnosis in 15% of cases of melanoma and only two-thirds of lesions overall were correctly diagnosed when compared to the histopathology (Grin et al. 1990). This does not take into account those that were not even biopsied.

In a recent study from St George's Hospital, London 120 lesions were excised either at the patient's request or for diagnostic purposes and clinical diagnoses compared with that of the pathologists (Curley et al. 1989). They highlighted the difficulty in distinguishing not only between dysplastic and banal naevi but also between naevi and other pigmented lesions. Small flat lesions were particularly difficult and three melanomas in the series were misdiagnosed by at least one observer. This important study bravely concluded that clinicians are only 50% correct when their diagnoses are compared with those of the histopathologist. The same authors also found that clinicians find it difficult to agree on the presence of signs in pigmented lesions and, in particular, whether lesions are irregular or not (Curley et al. 1990).

Surgeons with a special interest in melanoma can show that, for them, the diagnosis is easy (Griffiths et al. 1984) but it must be remembered that dermatologists tend to be referred a group of lesions that are diagnostically more difficult and contain the thinner melanomas (Rampen and Rumke 1988; Williams et al. 1991).

The dermatologist's nightmare is wrongly to reassure a patient with a melanoma. With the increasing pressure to recognize smaller and in-situ lesions anxiety will continue to rise. The safest solution would be to remove every pigmented lesion that is referred but this is not a practical solution. Because the diagnosis can often be difficult, there have been many tests and aids invented for the clinician to use.

Aids to Clinical Diagnosis

Nuclear Medicine Tests

No isotope study that has been tried, including injection of radioactive phosphorus (Brauer et al. 1960) and technetium-labelled antimelanoma antibodies (Rogers 1989) has been able to usefully detect cutaneous lesions.

Radiology 'Magnetic Resonance Imaging' Ultrasound

There is no adequate radiological technique for the diagnostic assessment of skin tumours (Hughes et al. 1987). Magnetic resonance imaging (MRI) has been recently tested in a few cases and theoretically shows promise since melanin can be made to be hyper-resonant and therefore appear as a bright area (Zemtsov 1989). This has yet to be evaluated with surface coils and it remains to be seen if it is of value in distinguishing melanoma from non-melanoma pigmented lesions.

High resolution ultrasound can be used for measuring tumour thickness prior to surgery (Reali et al. 1989) and there are reports that Doppler ultrasound can distinguish melanoma from basal cell papillomas by detecting a tumour hum even with a simple hand held device (Shukla and Hughes 1990). Laser Doppler is also being evaluated in some centres (Hughes et al. 1987). All of these techniques have the disadvantage of unproven benefit, cost and use restricted to specialist centres.

Surface Stripping

It has recently been reported that the technique of skin surface stripping can be 95% accurate in the diagnosis of melanomas (Pierard et al. 1989). The basis of this test is that a strip of plastic is glued to the top of a pigmented lesion using cyanoacrylate cement (Loctite 495). When this is "painlessly" pulled off, the stratum corneum comes with it and any atypical melanocytes present indicate abnormality. It has been advocated in the follow-up of patients with dysplastic naevus syndrome and may continue to show promise in the diagnosis of early lesions.

Surface Microscopy and the Dermatoscope

By covering a pigmented lesion with immersion oil and a glass slide and then examining it with a stereomicroscope the epidermis is rendered translucent and a new world of beautiful signs is revealed. A fine spider's web is seen at the periphery of melanocytic lesions but not at the edge of, for example, basal cell papillomas which are not derived from melanocytes. A whole range of subtle "dots" and "extensions" have been described which have their histological correlates (Soyer et al. 1989). These are supposed to help distinguish benign from malignant melanocytic lesions although no individual sign can be regarded as specific. In experienced hands up to 85% diagnostic accuracy can so far be achieved (MacKie 1971). Less expensive systems can be constructed based on standard single lens reflex cameras (Bahmer and Rohrer 1986) and an extremely portable and inexpensive hand-held device, the dermatoscope, is being purchased by a large number of UK dermatologists. There is clearly a learning curve to this technique and the interpretation is an extremely subjective art; nevertheless, many dermatologists feel reassured when holding a dermatoscope over a pigmented lesion.

Image Analysis

If a clinical photograph can be transferred onto a computer screen as a digital image then the computer recognizes it as a series of values, representing intensity of pigmentation, and co-ordinates, representing the spatial arrangement of the pigment. Image processing (IP) can enhance the two-dimensional characteristics

Table 4.3. Lesions studied

Histological type	Number of lesions
IDN	10
CN	20
BCP	15
NM	9
SMM	18
LM	19

IDN, intradermal naevus; CN, compound naevus; BCP, basal cell papilloma; NM, nodular melanoma; SMM, superficial malignant melanoma; LM, lentigo maligna melanoma.

of pigmented lesions for quantification by image analysis (IA). Thus the degree of pigmentation, pigment variation, the size, shape, irregularity and blurredness of the edge of pigmented lesions can all be measured and then assessed for their predictive value for diagnosing melanoma. Combinations of these parameters could, in theory be used for screening images and selecting those which have worrying features needing specialist clinical examination (Cascinelli et al. 1987). Techniques for quantifying some of the parameters that clinicians assess need to be developed to supplement standard IP methods. There are centres in Europe and the United States working separately on this subject. It is the author's view that we should pool our resources and particularly our databases of clinical photographs so that we can all refine our methods and share useful techniques.

The following is an account of some preliminary results from a collaborative study between the Blond McIndoe Centre for Medical Research, East Grinstead, and the School of Computer Science at Birmingham University.

In order that clinical photographs can meaningfully be compared in an objective way a calibrating scale showing a linear scale and a scale of neutral grey values across the spectrum from black to white must be included in the picture. We have developed a method of "normalization" of our images based on the standard Kodak step-wedge for controlling photographic development. Table 4.3 shows the breakdown of 91 lesions photographed prospectively using a Nikon FM2 with 105 mm Micronikkor macro lens adapted to incorporate a cut-down Kodak step-wedge and linear scale. The benign lesions were all removed for cosmetic rather than diagnostic purposes and the melanomas came from patients referred to either the Plastic Surgery Unit at East Grinstead, or the pigmented lesion clinics in Birmingham, Leicester, King's College or St George's Hospitals, London.

All lesions were first converted into analogue form using a Canon still-video camera and then captured as digital images on an Apple Macintosh IIci computer via a Neotech frame grabbing board. An IP software package, Optilab (Graftech UK), provided a comprehensive tool-box for processing and analysis.

The D,C,B,A system of Image Analysis in Melanoma

The American Academy ABCD system for the recognition of melanoma based on appearance contrasts with the emphasis in the UK on a history of change. Our preliminary results show that useful morphometric data can be extracted based on the ABCD system. By presenting the results in reverse order the best is saved to the last!

Diameter

Provided the number of pixels per millimetre on the screen is known the measurement of the longest diameter of the lesion is simple, accurate and automatic without the need for human judgement. Fig. 4.1 shows that all the melanomas were greater than 7 mm in maximum diameter. Thus this new cut-off point on the revised checklist holds well in this series yet one must caution against its use alone since in situ melanomas and early nodular (or papular) melanomas not analysed in this series would be missed. However, all but three lesions in this series were more than 5 mm so this cut-off point would be hopeless.

Colour

Analysis of pigment density and arrangement can be performed either on a "black and white" image which the computer recognizes as 256 levels of grey from black to white, or in the colour planes of red, green and blue each with 256 shades of intensity of colour. The human eye can only distinguish a maximum of 60 shades of grey and finds it difficult at times objectively to assess darkness of objects on different backgrounds. Fig. 4.2 displays the results for measuring how much darker than the surrounding skin the lesions were. It confirms our knowledge that lentigo maligna tend to be rather pale stains on the skin but disappointingly does not allow a cut-off point to be ruled to separate the melanomas from the benign lesions. It was anticipated that the darkest lesions would be the nodular melanomas but this was not the case.

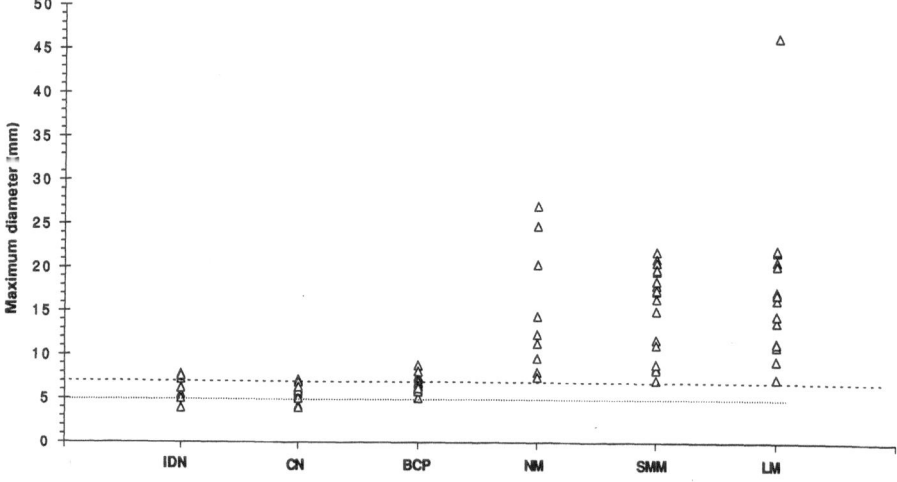

Fig. 4.1. Maximum diameter of the lesions studied. Lines are drawn at 5 mm and at 7 mm (the cut-off point on the revised check-list).

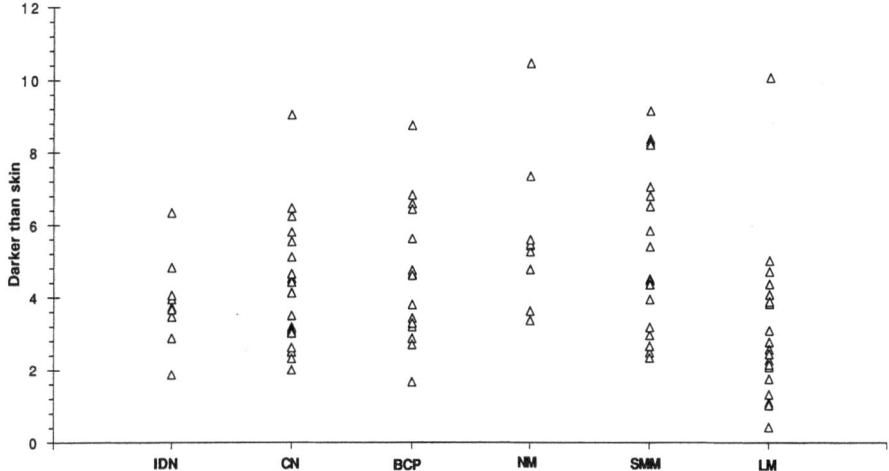

Fig. 4.2. Darkness of lesion in relation to the surrounding skin. The mean density of the skin tones (on a scale of 1–20) have been subtracted from the mean density of the lesion (on a scale of 1–20).

Intuitively one would anticipate that superficial malignant melanomas (SMMs) would exhibit the most variation in pigmentation. Fig. 4.3 shows that this assumption is only true for the minority of SMMs using the simple parameter of measuring the standard deviation of grey level intensity values. Fig. 4.4 is a histogram showing how the pigmentation in an SMM is made up of a series of peaks. This highlights the need for methods of assessing pigment distribution rather than crude overall variation. The information is there but needs to be extracted in a meaningful way.

The temptation to turn to analysis in the colour planes of red, green and blue seems logical but is thwarted by difficulties in standardization of colour and

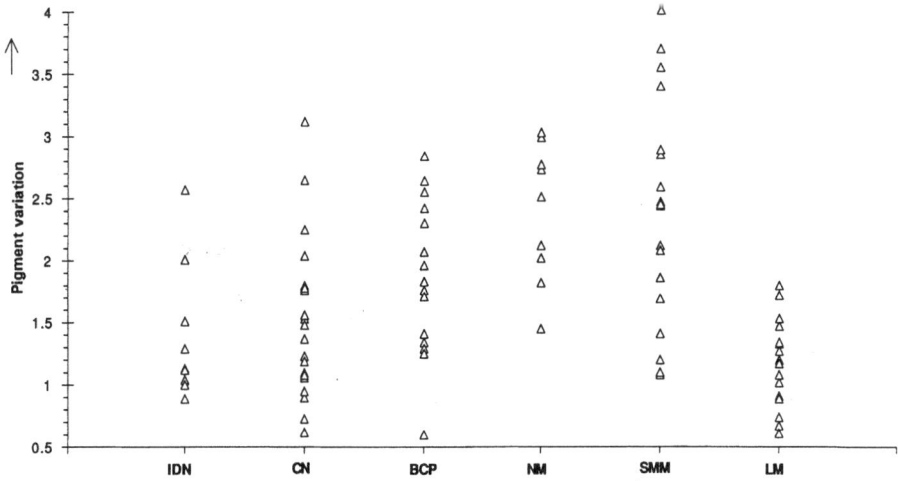

Fig. 4.3. Variation in pigmentation. The parameter of standard deviation of pigment intensity for each lesion has been plotted by histological type.

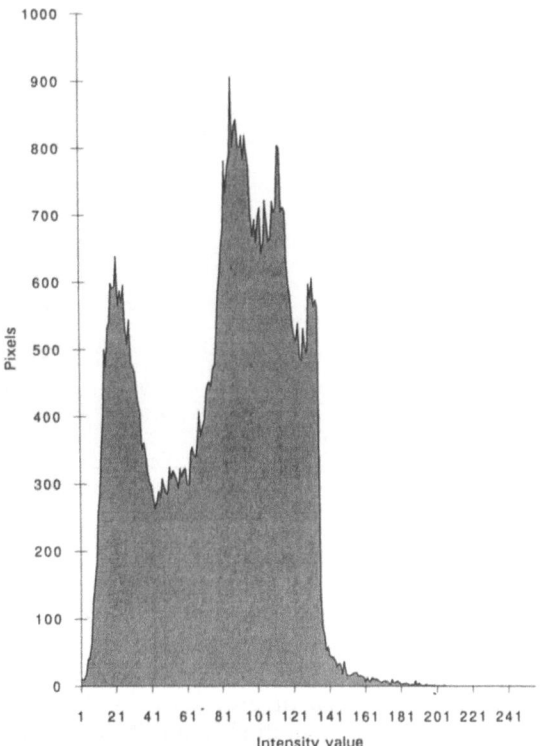

Fig. 4.4. Histogram of a superficial malignant melanoma. The number of pixels with each intensity value (on a scale of 0–255) has been plotted. Notice how there are several peaks which correspond to the multicoloured portions of the lesion.

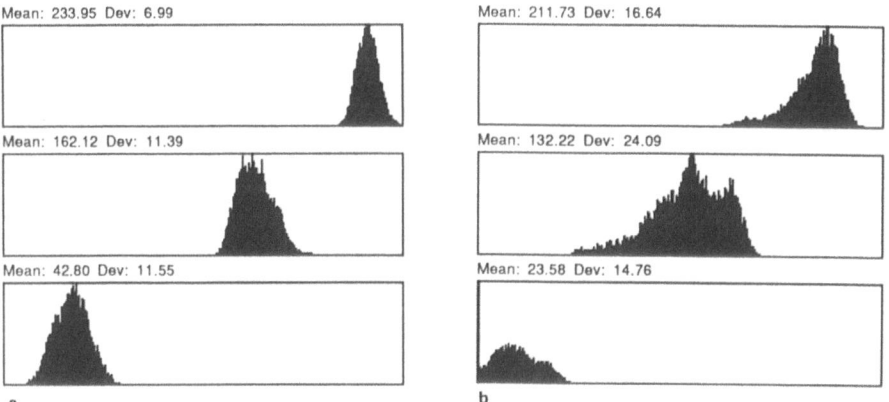

Fig. 4.5. **a** Histogram of the red, green and blue intensity values for an area of skin distant from an area of inflammation surrounding a nodular melanoma. **b** Histogram of the red, green and blue intensity values from an area of inflammation. Top, red; middle, green; bottom, blue.

colour balance. An enormous amount of numerical data can be generated and charts drawn to display this information. Interpretation is another matter which is presently beyond the scope of the author but perhaps less illusive to others. For instance inflammation appears to be due not just to an increase in intensity in the red spectrum, but rather, a relative change in the proportions of green and blue (Fig. 4.5).

Border

Clinically we tend to assess the border in two ways. The degree of sharpness or blurring and the regularity of the outline.

Edge Sharpness. IP techniques for quantifying the degree of sharpness of the edge are derived from the rate of change of pigmentation from one pixel to its neighbour on the screen. In artificial situations this works well but the presence of skin creases, hairs and reflected light make it necessary for techniques to be developed to filter out this "noise" before reliable conclusions can be drawn. When measuring the uniformity of edge sharpness in any particular lesion it is our impression that there is greater variation in melanomas than in benign lesions (Fig. 4.6). This seems to fit with one's clinical assessment. The polar co-ordinate transform is a computer method of unrolling the edge like unwinding a swiss-roll (Richter et al. 1991). It allows filtering of noise and may provide a more reliable method of assessing edge blurr.

Regularity of Outline. There has been much research on the quantification of irregularity of outline and shape in the chemical and powder industry. The degree of undulation of a perimeter can be measured using the principle of measuring the fractal dimension – a concept introduced by Mandelbrot (1967). He discovered

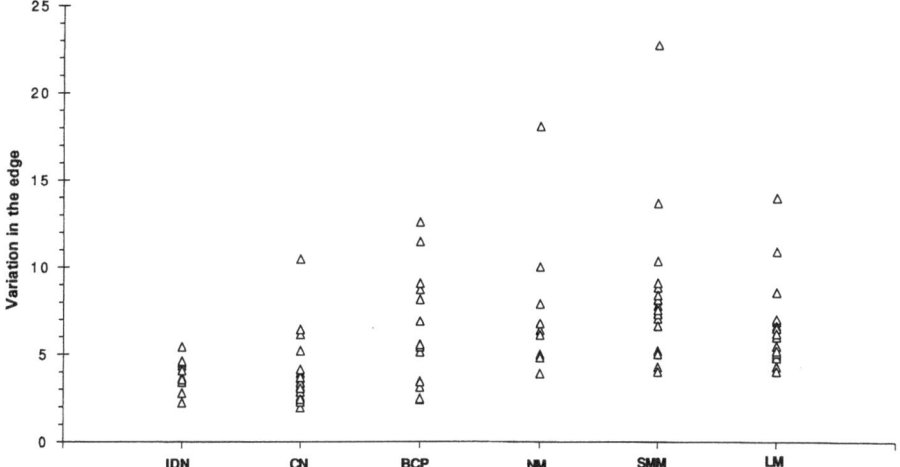

Fig. 4.6. Variation in the edge. Using the Sobel filter for estimating the rate of change of intensity values the degree of edge sharpness can be estimated. This chart shows the variation in sharpness of the edge of histological types.

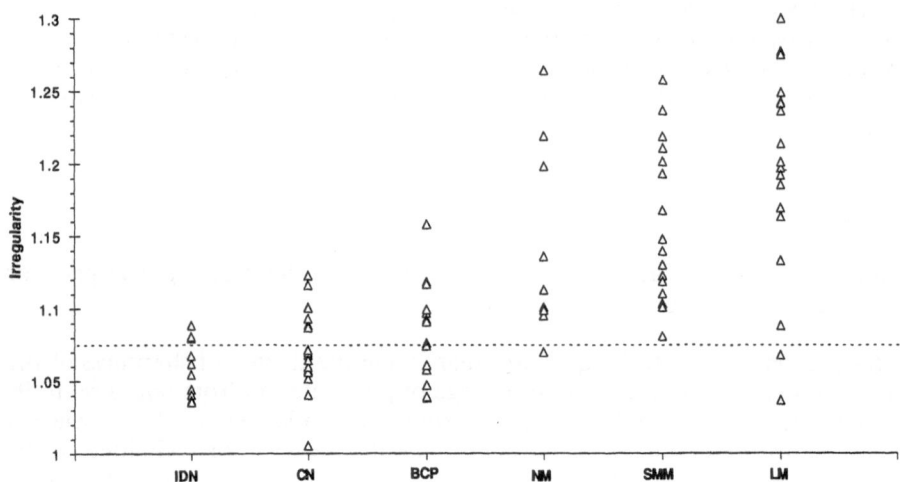

Fig. 4.7. Textural fractal dimensions by histological type. The degree of irregularity increases along the vertical axis. The dotted line marks the value found in a previous study to separate the most irregular from the most regular. Most of the melanomas are irregular using this parameter.

that if the coast-line of Great Britain was measured with a pair of dividers, then the length of the perimeter obtained got smaller as the width of the jaws on the dividers became wider. A plot of perimeter measured versus step-length yields a straight line whose slope is termed the "fractal dimension". It was further found that with very small "step-lengths" the fine details of the perimeter could be quantified as the "textural fractal" but once the step-length reached a critical size the overall undulations of the perimeter were quantified as the "structural fractal" (Kaye 1989). The textural and structural fractals for the pigmented lesions studied were measured using the method described by Flook (1978) and are shown in Figs 4.7 and 4.8 respectively. In a previous study, when computer-ized IA was compared with the ability of British dermatologists to distinguish benign pigmented lesions from melanoma based on their silhouette, cut-off points between the most regular lesions (assumed to be benign) and irregular lesions (assumed to be melanomas) were found (Hall et al. 1991). Using the same criteria on this prospectively collected data set, textural fractals (Fig. 4.7) were very sensitive (93.5%) but not very specific (62.2%) whereas structural fractals (Fig. 4.8) were less sensitive (76%) but more specific (84.4%). Thus quantification of irregularity of outline appears to be an extremely useful way of separating melanoma from non-melanoma pigmented lesions.

Asymmetry of Shape

In quantifying shape we have not looked at asymmetry but at methods that express the degree of matching to an ellipse, since one might expect that benign lesions would tend to be elliptical or circular whereas malignant ones will be less regular in shape. A number of computer methods exist for the measurement of circularity most of which are inappropriate for use in pigmented lesions. The measurement

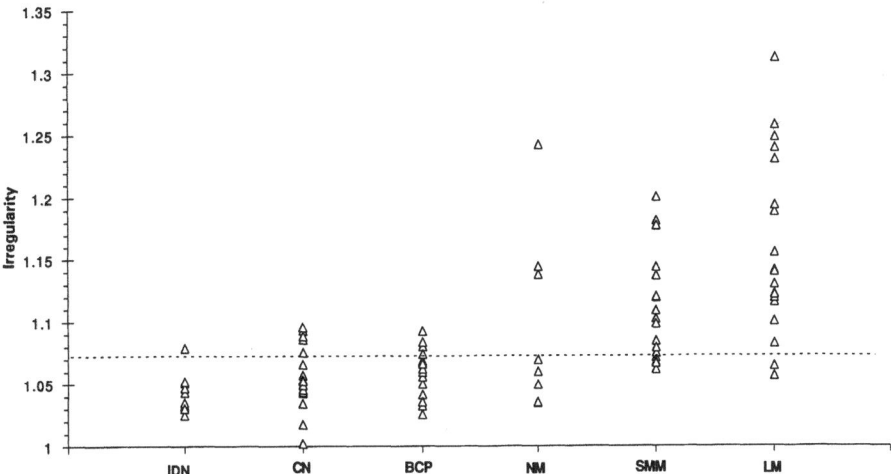

Fig. 4.8. Structural fractal dimensions by histological type. The degree of irregularity increases along the vertical axis.

of "bulkiness" as described by Medalia (1970) is a method of quantification of shape which appears to correlate well with the way in which the British dermatologists assessed the irregularity of silhouettes in the previously mentioned study. The digital image of a lesion can be separated from its background skin tones by the computer using a "thresholding" IP technique. The image is converted into binary format so that every pixel on the screen is regarded as belonging to either the lesion, or the background. The centre of the lesion is found and an equivalent ellipse calculated whose long and short axes bear a relationship to the positions in space of every point in the lesion relative to the centre. The ratio of the area of the equivalent ellipse divided by the area of the lesion is the "bulkiness score". A circular and an elliptical lesion will be expected to have a bulkiness of 1 (since both will have equivalent ellipses identical with the original), so irregularity increases with the bulkiness score. Fig. 4.9 shows the bulkiness score for the lesions in this study. The sensitivity for bulkiness using the same cut-off point as in the previous study was high (89%) as was the specificity (86.7%).

Combination of Image Analysis Parameters

In the previous study 93% of melanomas could be screened from non-melanoma pigmented lesions by combining the fractal dimensions and bulkiness scores as a series of filters with a specificity of 91%. Using the same cut-points, combining all three parameters separates all but one melanoma, including an amelanotic melanoma (sensitivity 97.8%) and does not falsely identify any of the benign lesions as malignant (specificity 100%). The missed lesion was a nodular melanoma which had a maximum diameter of 30 mm and which happened to have the darkest overall mean intensity value compared with the neighbouring skin.

These results are very encouraging but need to be evaluated on a larger data set

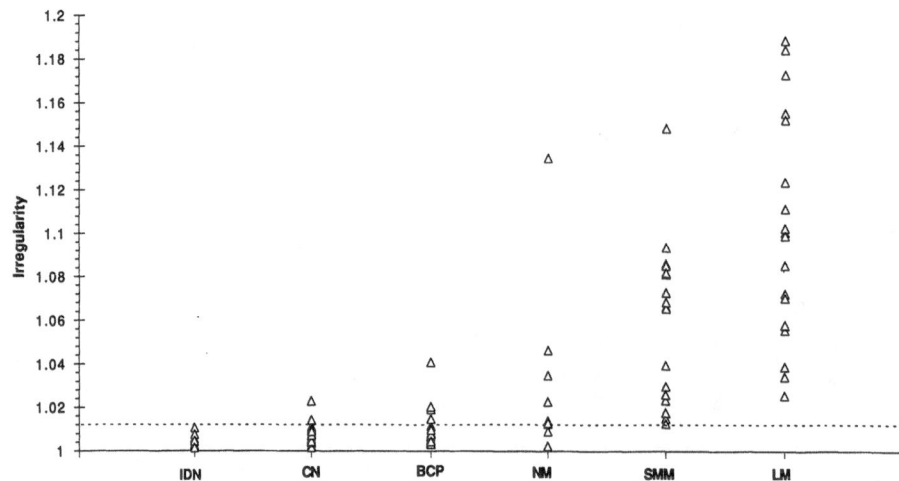

Fig. 4.9. Bulkiness score by histological types. The degree of irregularity increases along the vertical axis.

which should include all types of pigmented lesions seen in pigmented lesion clinics in the proportions of melanoma to non-melanoma expected. Further computer methods to extract the available information in meaningful ways to quantify edge sharpness, pigment variation and surface texture and a better understanding of colour can only improve the results. The possibility of an objective screening tool based on image analysis of pigmented lesions is not beyond our reach.

References

Ackerman BA (1985) Malignant melanoma in situ: the flat curable stage of malignant melanoma. Pathology 17:298–300

Bahmer FA, Rohrer C (1986) Rapid and simple macrophotography of the skin. Br J Dermatol 114:135–136

Becker SW (1954) Pitfalls in the diagnosis and treatment of melanoma. Arch Dermatol 69:11–30

Brauer EW, Kopf AW, Witten VH, Berman M, Cave V (1960) Radioactive phosphorus in the in vivo diagnosis of melanoma of the skin. JAMA 172:1753–1758

Cameron JRJ (1968) Melanoma of the skin. Clinical account of a series of 209 malignant melanomas of the skin. J R Coll Surg Edinb 13:235–254

Cascinelli N, Ferrario M, Tonelli T et al. (1987) A possible new tool for the diagnosis of melanoma: the computer. J Am Acad Dermatol 16:361–367

Clark WH, From I, Bernardino EA, Mihm MC (1969) The histogenesis and biologic behaviour of primary malignant melanomas of the skin. Cancer Res 29:705–727

Curley RK, Cook MG, Fallowfield ME, Marsden RA (1989) Accuracy in clinically evaluating pigmented lesions. Br Med J 299:16–18

Curley RK, Fallowfield ME, Cook MG, Marsden RA (1990) The clinical features of dysplastic naevi: interobserver agreement and correlation with histology. Br J Dermatol 123:119–120

Doherty VR, MacKie RM (1986) Reasons for poor prognosis in British patients with cutaneous malignant melanoma. Br Med J 292:987–989

Doherty VR, MacKie RM (1988) Experience of a public education program on early detection of cutaneous malignant melanoma. Br Med J 297:388–391

du Vivier AWP, Higgins EM (1991) Clinical recognition of early invasive malignant melanoma. Letter. Br Med J 302:49–50

du Vivier AWP, William HC, Brett JV, Higgins E (1990) How do malignant melanomas present and does this correlate with the 7 point checklist? Br J Dermatol 123(suppl):39

Fitzsimmons CP, MacKie RM, Wilson PD (1984) A study of total number and distribution of melanocytic naevi in a British population. Br J Dermatol 3(suppl):9

Flook AG (1978) The use of dilation logic on the Quantimet to achieve fractal dimension characterisation of texture and structured profiles. Powder Technol 21:295–298

Graham-Brown RAC, Osbourne JE, London SP et al. (1990) The initial effects on workload and outcome of a public education campaign on early diagnosis and treatment of malignant melanoma in Leicestershire. Br J Dermatol 122:53–59

Griffiths RW, Briggs JC, Hiles RW (1984) Clinical diagnostic accuracy in the management of primary stage I cutaneous malignant melanoma in a plastic surgery unit. Bristol MedicoChirurgical Journal April:55–60

Grin CM, Kopf AW, Welkovich B, Bart RS, Levenstein MJ (1990) Accuracy in the clinical diagnosis of malignant melanoma. Arch Dermatol 126:763–767

Hall PN, Keefe M, Allen J, Claridge E (1991) Distinguishing benign pigmented lesions from melanoma. Melanoma '91 (Poster)

Higgins E, du Vivier AWP (1991) Malignant melanoma – a review: early diagnosis is the key. Br J Clin Pract 45:109–115

Higgins EM, Todd P, Hall PN, Murthi R, du Vivier AWP (1991) The predictive value of the seven-point checklist in the assessment of benign pigmented lesions. Br J Dermatol 125(suppl):19

Hughes BR, Black D, Srivastva A (1987) Comparison of techniques for the non-invasive assessment of skin tumours. Clin Exp Dermatol 12:108–111

Kaye BH (1989) A random walk through fractal dimensions. VCH publishers, New York

Keefe M, Dick DC, Wakeel RA (1990a) A study of the value of the seven-point checklist in distinguishing benign pigmented lesions from melanoma. Clin Exp Dermatol 15:167–171

Keefe M, White JE, Perkins P (1990b) Nodular melanomas in the over 50 age group: the next target for health education. Br J Dermatol 123(suppl):59

Koh HK, Lew RA, Prout MN (1989) Screening for melanoma/skin cancer: theoretic and practical considerations. J Am Acad Dermatol 20:159–172

MacKie RM (1971) An aid to the pre-operative assessment of pigmented lesions of the skin. Br J Dermatol 16:407–410

MacKie RM (1985) An illustrated guide to the recognition of early malignant melanoma. University Department of Dermatology, Glasgow

MacKie RM (1989) Malignant melanoma. A guide to early diagnosis. University Department of Dermatology, Glasgow

MacKie RM (1990) Clinical recognition of early invasive malignant melanoma. Editorial. Br Med J 301:1005–1006

Mandelbrot BB (1967) How long is the coast of Britain, statistical self-similarity and fractional dimension. Science 155:636–638

McMullan FH, Hubener LF (1956) Malignant melanoma. A statistical review of clinical and histological diagnoses. Arch Dermatol 74:618–619

Medalia AI. (1970) Dynamic shape factors of particles. Powder Technol 4:117–138

Pierard GE, Pierard-Franchimont C, Estrada JA et al. (1989) Cyanoacrylate skin surface stripping: an improved approach for distinguishing dysplatic nevi from malignant melanomas. J Cutan Pathol 16:180–182

Rampen FHJ, Rumke P (1988) Referral pattern and accuracy of clinical diagnosis of cutaneous melanoma. Acta Derm Venereol 68:61–64

Reali UM, Santucci M, Paoli G, Chirugi C (1989) The use of high resolution ultrasound in preoperative evaluation of cutaneous melanoma thickness. Tumori 75:452–455

Richter J, Hall PN, Claridge E (1991) Computer assisted measurement of edge blur in pigmented lesions. Melanoma '91 (Poster)

Rogers GS (1989) Melanoma update. Advances in diagnostic technique. J Dermatol Surg Oncol 15:605–607

Sagebiel RW (1979) Histopathology of borderline and early malignant melanoma. Am J Surg Pathol 3:543–552

Shukla VK, Hughes LE (1989) Differential diagnosis of subungual melanoma from a surgical point of view. Br J Surg 76:1156–1160

Shukla VK, Hughes LE (1990) Naevi and melanomas. Surgery 79:1888–1895
Sober AJ (1985) The changing mole. JAMA 253:1612–1613
Sondergaard K (1985) Biological behaviour of cutaneous malignant melanomas. Pathology 17:255–257
Soyer HP, Smolle J, Hodl S et al. (1989) Surface microscopy. A new approach to the diagnosis of cutaneous pigmented tumours. Am J Dermatopathol 11:1–10
Swerdlow M (1952) Nevi: a problem of misdiagnosis. Am J Clin Pathol 22:1054–1060
Todd P, Higgins E, Humphries S, du Vivier A (1991) A study of the clinical and pathological features of in-situ melanoma. Br J Dermatol 125(suppl):18
Walton RG, Jacobs AG, Cox AJ (1976) Pigmented lesions of the new born. Br J Dermatol 95:389
Whitehead SM, Wroughton MA (1988) Education campaign on early detection of malignant melanoma. Br Med J 297:620–621
Williams HC, Smith D, du Vivier AWP (1990) Evaluation of public education campaigns in cutaneous melanoma: the King's College Hospital experience. Br J Dermatol 123:85–92
Williams HC, Smith D, du Vivier AWP (1991) Melanoma: differences between general surgeons and dermatologists. Int J Dermatol 30:257–261
Zemtsov A, Lorig R, Bergfield W, Bailin P, Ng TC (1989) Magnetic resonance imaging of cutaneous melanocytic lesions. J Dermatol Surg Oncol 15:854–858

5   Familial Melanoma

Julia A. Newton

Although the incidence of melanoma is increasing (now 10 per 100000 in the UK (Roberts 1990)) it is still relatively uncommon so that clustering of melanoma in families is always significant and should be explored. Families may share common risk factors for melanoma such as red hair, freckles and a tendency to burn in the sun. They may also have a shared lifestyle, particularly in terms of sun exposure which is an important risk factor for melanoma (Evans et al. 1988). Familial melanoma may, therefore, occur due to these shared risk factors especially in areas of higher incidence such as Australia.

There are, however, distinct family cancer syndromes in which there is a genetic predisposition to melanoma. The family cancer syndromes are probably very much more common than had been previously supposed and are not yet fully delineated. Areas of overlap may exist. However, it is probable that genetic predisposition to melanoma may occur in at least four forms. The best described is the atypical mole syndrome, about which this review is predominantly concerned. Melanomas may also occur as a second malignancy in familial retinoblastoma and in two family cancer syndromes known as Lynch type II (colon cancer, endometrial cancer, breast cancer, pancreas cancer and mela- noma) and the Li-Fraumeni syndrome (bilateral early onset breast carcinoma, soft tissue sarcomas, gliomas, melanomas and lung carcinoma). The occurrence of melanoma in the Li-Fraumeni syndrome is better established than in Lynch type II family cancer syndrome.

The most clearly defined familial form of melanoma (the FAMMM atypical mole syndrome, dysplastic naevus syndrome or B-K mole syndrome) was first described by Wallace Clark (Clark et al. 1978). He studied two families with a high incidence of melanoma and found that the individuals with melanoma also had unusual moles. These moles have come to be known as dysplastic naevi, having a characteristic clinical and (when biopsied) histological appearance. They tend to be predominantly flat and larger than most moles with an ill-defined blurred margin. There is colour variation and sometimes irregularity of the edge. Histological changes may be described as architectural (with elongation of the rete pegs and lentiginous hyperplasia of melanocytes), cytological (nuclear atypia usually of a mild to moderate severity) and stromal (collagen condensation, lymphocytic infiltration and vascular hyperplasia) (Elder 1988). Clark has described the dysplastic naevus as a naevus representing aberrant differentiation and as such represents one stage in stepwise tumour progression (Clark et al. 1984). In familial melanoma the presence of such moles may serve as markers for susceptibility to melanoma as well as representing putative premalignant lesions. In one pathological study 32.4% of 500 superficial spreading melanomas, showed evidence of residual dysplastic naevus (Black 1988). The vast majority of these moles, however, are mature end-stage lesions which ultimately regress as do common moles.

The atypical mole syndrome (AMS) is characterized by the presence of the atypical naevi described above but there is no precise definition of phenotype. Since 1976 it has been recognized that small numbers of dysplastic naevi occur in the general population – a figure of 8%–9% of the population being found both in Europe (Curley 1989) and in New Zealand (Cooke et al. 1989) so there has been considerable concern about the difficulties of the clinical recognition of the condition. The situation has been further exacerbated by disagreement about the specificity of the histological features of dysplasia (Clark and Ackerman 1989). Even among affected members of families there appears to be considerable variation in the types and numbers of moles present.

Detailed clinical studies are currently taking place at the Royal London Hospital to document the types, numbers and distribution of naevi in the AMS.

In an affected child the first evidence of abnormality is usually the development of increased numbers of banal naevi at about the age of 5 to 10 years. Subsequently slightly pink, larger naevi become obvious, particularly on the scalp. The phenotype is usually fully established by the age of 20 (Crutcher 1988). An affected adult should be recognized not just by looking for the "classical" appearance of a dysplastic naevus but by considering various aspects of his phenotype (Table 5.1). Two or three clinically dysplastic naevi may be considered "normal" in the absence of a family history of melanoma, but would be viewed differently if the total mole count was high (e.g. over 100 greater than 2 mm in diameter) or if there were moles on the buttocks or breasts. It is perhaps similar to an assessment of a child with four café au lait spots. The dermatologist will be reassuring without a family history of neurofibromatosis, a little more circumspect if the family history is positive. Similarly if the child has axillary freckling then the café au lait spots would have much greater significance.

The AMS phenotype is usually easy to recognize if all the clinical features in Table 5.1 are considered together. The moles, if counted, usually number in excess of 100 greater than 2 mm in diameter. The distribution of the moles is abnormal being present on the buttocks, ears, hands and feet and scalp. The appearance of the moles is usually abnormal but it is important to stress that in

Table 5.1. Aspects of phenotype to be considered in making a clinical diagnosis of the atypical mole syndrome

1. Increased total mole count for that age
2. Significant numbers of moles on covered skin
3. Significant numbers of moles on dorsum and lateral borders of the feet and hands
4. The presence of atypical or classically dysplastic moles
5. The presence of iris freckles or moles
6. Melanomas especially if multiple or in unusual sites, e.g. buttocks, breast or scalp

our experience not all patients have moles which conform to be classical dysplastic naevus as described by Clark. It is not uncommon, for example, to see a parent with numerous but normal looking naevi and melanoma and the child with dysplastic naevi. We consider large numbers of iris freckles/naevi to be a very valuable sign of the AMS. Finally, one should be very suspicious if melanomas are either multiple or occur in unusual sites such as on the breasts and scalp.

In normal individuals the numbers of moles reach their peak at about the age of 35 years and subsequently the moles disappear so that 70 or 80 year olds have few or none. In the AMS the tendency to produce moles is exaggerated so that individuals continue to develop new dysplastic naevi until much later. The futility of "prophylactic excision" of these moles is illustrated by a case report of a 31-year-old with numerous new histologically confirmed dysplastic naevi who seven years previously had had all his naevi (over 150) "prophylactically excised" (Barnes and Nordlund 1987). Nonetheless, eventually the number of moles does reduce and an affected individual of 70 or 80 years may only have biopsy scars as evidence of their previous appearance.

A clinical diagnosis may be easier when the individual's first degree relatives are screened. The variation in expression of this condition is such that not infrequently a clinical impression may be strengthened or weakened by finding evidence of the AMS or absence of the AMS respectively in relatives.

When naevi look very atypical clinically, particularly if there is marked colour variation (suggesting junctional activity) or if the lesion is changing then it is our practice to biopsy. The criteria for biopsy are, therefore, the same as for any pigmented lesion clinic. The aim is to detect and remove early any superficial spreading melanomas. It is not our practice to excise naevi to confirm our diagnosis of the AMS. There is sufficient histological overlap between benign and clinically dysplastic naevi to make this in our view unhelpful.

Genetics

Most groups currently accept that the AMS is caused by an autosomal dominant gene although with rather variably incomplete penetrance. The Leiden group, for example, have found penetrance in their families to be only 30%–40% depending on whether one considers the occurrence of melanomas or dysplastic naevi (Bergman et al. 1986). Analysis of mutation rate estimates and the presence of AMS phenotype in sporadic cases in whom the risk of melanoma appears to be less than in familial AMS has led some authors to suggest that the mode of inheritance may actually be polygenic (Traupe et al. 1989; Traupe and Happle 1990). The rare occurrence of quadrantic distribution of AMS, however, supports the concept of a single gene (Sterry and Christophers 1988). The situation remains unclear and controversial.

Genetic linkage studies are in progress in several centres now assuming that the AMS is truly autosomal dominant. Bale et al. (1989) suggested that the gene for AMS was on the short arm of chromosome 1 (1p36) but unfortunately this has not been confirmed in other centres (Van Haeringen et al. 1989; Cannon-Albright et al. 1990). Genetic heterogeneity may prove to be the explanation of this disparity: as yet the situation is controversial and unclear. Linkage studies continue, made difficult because of incomplete penetrance and variable phenotypes.

Karyotypic studies of melanoma tissue may give a clue to the site of the AMS gene. These have shown that deletions and translocations are most common on chromosome 1, 6, 7 and 11 and, therefore, these may be the most likely sites for the AMS gene. Laboratory studies designed to detect abnormal responses to UV light in families with the AMS have produced some evidence for DNA sensitivity in that there was delay in starting to repair DNA after UV exposure (Ramsay et al. 1982). Normal DNA repair synthesis, however, has been demonstrated (Ringborg et al. 1980; Ramsay et al. 1982) which appears to exclude a variant of xeroderma pigmentosum as a cause of the AMS.

Estimates of Risk of Melanoma

It is desirable to give patients with the AMS phenotype an estimate of their risk of developing a melanoma, particularly because it may be very variable. Kraemer has classified the AMS into groups A, B, C, D1 and D2 (Kraemer et al. 1983) (Table 5.2) and has estimated that the relative risk of an individual with the AMS alone and no family history may only be 7. The relative risk for an individual at the other extreme with dysplastic naevi from a family with two previous melanomas, however, is probably around 500. We have found Kraemer's classification useful in the clinical setting. Full evaluation of the system in risk estimation, is however not complete. It is valuable to put a relative risk of 7 in perspective: every red-haired individual for example has a relative risk of 3.

Table 5.2. Kraemer's classification of the dysplastic naevus syndrome with gross estimates of relative risk for melanoma. Type C may represent new mutations so that in time offspring may develop the AMS and reclassification to type D1 would be necessary

Group	Relative risk	Phenotype
A B	7 to 27	Dysplastic naevi individual alone Familial dysplastic naevi
C		Dysplastic naevi and melanoma in the individual alone
D1		Familial dysplastic naevi and one melanoma in family
D2	500	Familial DNS and at least two melanomas

Management of AMS Patients

Once the diagnosis of the AMS has been made, it is important to screen all first-degree relatives and if there is a family history of melanoma, selected second degree relatives too. Although time consuming this is important, especially with a family history of melanoma, because of the partial penetrance of the gene. Bergman et al. (1986) found 12 unsuspected melanomas by screening 243 family members of six families. Screening usually starts at 12 years of age. We, however, do see children earlier if the parents are worried. It also serves the function of reinforcing advice about the importance of sun avoidance in childhood.

The early detection of further melanomas must be facilitated by patient education about what to look for, and by instituting proper follow-up. In our unit families are usually seen together and are taught about the clinical appearances of moles and melanoma in groups and using family members' own moles as examples. Initial follow-up for one year is at four-monthly intervals. In many individuals with stable moles, who are competent at self examination, the frequency may then be reduced to annual follow-up but with very ready access to clinic if the patient is concerned. Patients with unstable moles should be seen at least every four months. Some units use extensive photography in patient follow-up (MacKie et al. 1983; Batimer and Rohser 1986). In our unit the most atypical naevi are marked and photographed using a camera with a ring flash, fixed focus and calibration plate which is placed onto the skin around the mole. The transparencies are then available for projection in clinic.

Education about sun avoidance is also given. Patients are encouraged never to sunbathe and particular attention is given to advice about children under the age of 15. Case control studies in sporadic melanoma have shown that severe sunburn in childhood is a risk factor for malignant melanoma and it is, therefore, likely to be similarly important in the AMS.

Non-Melanoma Malignancy in the AMS Families

A subset of the Leiden families studied by Wilma Bergman have been shown to have an increased frequency of gastrointestinal tract neoplasms particularly carcinoma of the pancreas. A further group had an increased tendency to ocular melanoma (Bergman et al. 1990) but this was not confirmed by studies in the USA (Greene et al. 1987).

The possible association between eye and cutaneous melanoma is particularly interesting. There have been several case reports of eye and cutaneous melanoma occurring in individuals (e.g. Bellet et al. 1980; Oosterhuis et al. 1982) but the link has been decribed as coincidental (Greene et al. 1983). We are, therefore, in the process of screening sequential eye melanoma patients attending oncology clinics at Moorfields and St Bartholomew's Hospitals, under the care of Mr John Hungerford, for the presence of abnormal moles. Over 200 patients have so far been screened of which 6% have the AMS phenotype. One patient had unsuspected melanomas at screening. Screening of relatives of these individuals is currently taking place and it is, therefore, not possible to specify in how many patients this is familial AMS. Fig. 5.1, however, illustrates two small pedigrees in which familial AMS was seen. It is clear, therefore, that AMS patients may develop eye melanoma, but the incidence is as yet unclear. Ocular screening of patients with cutaneous melanoma would seem to be indicated but as yet there are no pointers as to whether selected patients are at particular risk.

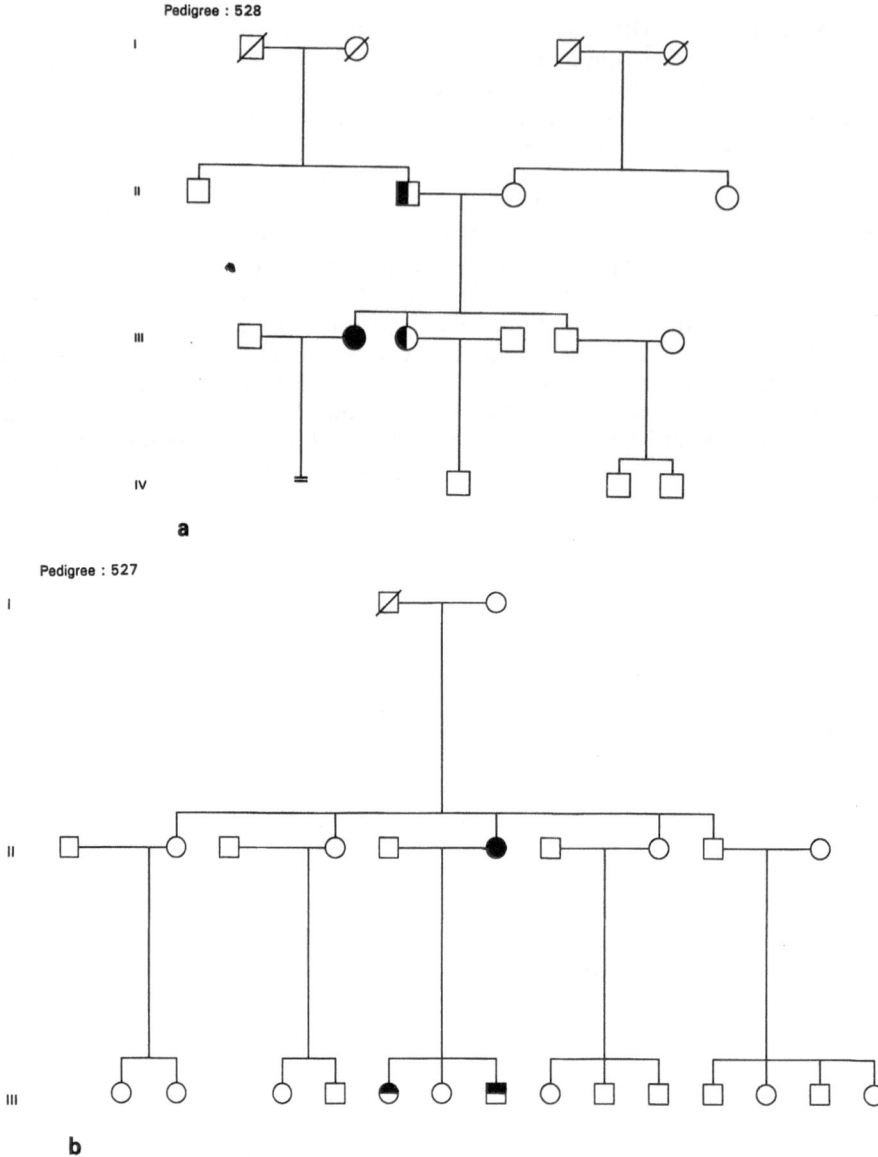

Fig. 5.1. Two pedigrees illustrating the occurrence of eye and cutaneous melanoma in the AMS. **a** The AMS phenotype; **b** AMS skin and eye melanoma.

Conclusions

The presence of large numbers of moles atypical in appearance and distribution typifies the atypical mole syndrome. The syndrome may occur in one individual alone or in an autosomal dominant fashion in their family. The presence of this phenotype indicates an increased risk of melanoma although the risk varies according to the presence or absence of a family history. The classification devised by Kraemer et al. (1983) works well in estimating risk of melanomas.

The diagnosis of the syndrome is essentially clinical necessitating the consideration of various aspects of phenotype such as total mole count, distribution, clinical appearance of the moles and the age of onset, site and number of melanomas. It is always helpful to screen first-degree relatives and second degree if there is a family history of "moleyness" or melanoma.

Small numbers of clinically and sometimes histologically dysplastic naevi may occur in normal individuals. The vast majority of these probably regress as do totally banal naevi although a low percentage will result in a melanoma (Black 1988). Those patients should be questioned about a family history of increased numbers of moles and melanoma. They should also be thoroughly examined for the presence of other signs of the syndrome: increased total mole count, iris freckles etc. In the absence of either a family history of these additional clinical features then it is unlikely that these individuals have "the syndrome". Common sense advice about sun avoidance and self examination should be given. It is important to distinguish this from the AMS syndrome.

Many authors are unhappy about the use of the term "dysplastic naevus syndrome" for this condition partly because the histological appearances of the atypical naevi are not dysplastic in the true sense of the word (Rywlin 1989). There has also been considerable unease among pathologists about the implications of reporting a naevus as "dysplastic". The situation may be improved if it is recognized that dysplastic naevi can occur normally in the general population and what is important is the recognition of the full phenotype and family history. Some patients from melanoma families do not have "classically dysplastic" naevi. It is, therefore, probably better to abandon the term dysplastic naevus syndrome in favour of the atypical mole syndrome.

References

Bale SJ, Dracopoli NC, Tucker MA et al. (1989) Mapping the gene for hereditary cutaneous malignant melanoma – dysplastic nevus to chromosome 1p. N Engl J Med 320:1367–1372

Barnes LM, Nordlund JJ (1987). The natural history of dysplastic nevi. Arch Dermatol 123:1059–1061.

Batimer FA, Rohser C (1986) Rapid and simple macro-photography of the skin. Br J Dermatol 114:135–136

Bellet RE, Shields JA, Soll DB, Bernardino EA (1980) Primary choroidal and cutaneous melanomas occurring in a patient with the B-K mole syndrome phenotype. Am J Ophthalmol 89:567–570

Bergman W, Palan A, Went LN (1986) Clinical and genetic studies in six Dutch patients with the DNS. Ann Hum Genet 50:249–258

Bergman W, Watson P, de Jong J. Lynch HT, Fusaro RM (1990) Systemic cancer and the FAMMM syndrome. Br J Cancer 61:932–936

Black WC (1988) Residual dysplastic and other nevi in superficial spreading melanoma. Cancer 62:163–173

Cannon-Albright LA, Goldgar DE, Wright EC et al. (1990) Evidence against the reported linkage of the cutaneous melanoma – dysplastic nevus syndrome locus to chromosone 1p36. Am J Hum Genet 46:912–918

Clark WH, Elder DE, Guerry IV D et al. (1984) A study of tumour progression: the precursor lesions of superficial spreading and nodular melanoma. Hum Pathol 15:1147–1165

Clark WH, Ackerman AB (1989) An exchange of views regarding the dysplastic nevus controversy. Semin Dermatol 18:229–250

Clark WM, Reimer RR, Greene M et al. (1978) Origin of familial malignant melanomas from heritable melanocytic lesions: "the B.K. mole syndrome". Arch Dermatol 114:732–738

Cooke KR, Spears GFS, Elder DE, Greene MH (1989) Dysplastic nevi in a population based study. Cancer 63: 1240–1244

Crutcher WA (1988) The dysplastic nevus and its clinical management. Adv Dermatol 3:187–204

Curley R (1989) Oral communication. 2nd International Conference on Melanoma. Venice

Elder DE (1988) Dysplastic nevi: their significance and management. Pigmentation disorders. Dermatol Clin 6:257–269

Evans RD, Kopf AW, Lew RA et al. (1988) Risk factors for the development of malignant melanoma – I: review of case control studies. J Dermatol Surg Oncol 14:393–408

Greene MH, Sanders RJ, Chu FC et al. (1983) The familial occurrence of cutaneous melanoma, intra-ocular melanoma and the dysplastic nevus syndrome. Am J Ophthalmol 96:238–245

Greene MH, Tucker MA, Clark WH et al. (1987) Hereditary melanoma and the dysplastic nevus syndrome: the risk of cancers other than melanoma. J Am Acad Dermatol 16:792–797

Kraemer KH, Greene MH, Tarone R et al. (1983) Dysplastic nevi and cutaneous melanoma risk. Lancet ii:1076–1077

MacKie RM, English J, Ashworth J et al. (1983) Managing the dysplastic nevus. Lancet ii:1249–1250

Oosterhuis JA, Went LN, Lynch HT (1982) Primary choroidal and cutaneous melanomas, bilateral choroidal melanomas and familial occurrence of melanomas. Br J Ophthalmol 66:230–233

Ramsay RG, Glen, P, Imray FP et al. (1982) Familial melanoma associated with dominant ultraviolet radiation sensitivity. Cancer Res 42:2909–2912

Ringborg V, Legerlof B, Lambert B (1980) Normal UV induced DNA repair synthesis in peripheral leukocytes from patients with malignant melanoma of the skin. J Invest Dermatol 74:72–73

Roberts DL (1990) Malignant melanoma in West Glamorgan: increasing incidence and improving prognosis 1986–1988. Clin Exp Dermatol 15:406–409

Rywlin AM (1989). Some remarks on dysplasia. Am J Dermatopathol 11:390–391

Sterry W, Christophers E (1988) Quadrant distribution of dysplastic nevus syndrome. Arch Dermatol 124:926–929

Traupe H, Happle R (1990) The dysplastic nevus syndrome is not a dichotomic but a continuous phenotype. Am J Med Genet 35:295–296

Traupe H, Macher E, Hamm H, Happle R (1989) Mutation rate estimates are not compatible with autosomal dominant inheritance of the dysplastic nevus syndrome. Am J Med Genet 32:155–157

Van Haeringen A, Bergman W, Nelen MR et al. (1989) Exclusion of the dysplastic naevus syndrome (DNS) locus from the short arm of chromosome 1 by linkage studies in Dutch families. Genomics 5:61–64

6   The Histological Diagnosis of Cutaneous Melanoma.

W. J. Mooi and T. Krausz

Cutaneous melanoma, although essentially a single entity – a malignant tumour of cutaneous melanocytes – exhibits a wide spectrum of histological appearances. Some tumours are densely cellular, with a compact and nodular pattern of growth, whereas others consist of a diffuse and ill-defined paucicellular spindle-cell proliferation which may be difficult to delineate from the surrounding tissues. Cell types vary from polygonal or rounded to elongated and dendritic; in some melanomas, the tumour cells show only very mild pleomorphism, in others, they are bizarre and exceedingly pleomorphic. Some tumours retain a very superficial growth pattern for many years, whereas others rapidly form masses which deeply penetrate the skin and underlying tissues.

Because of these differences, numerous clinicopathological subtypes of cutaneous melanoma have been proposed in the literature; however, unfortunately, a compilation of these different subtypes does not result in an internally consistent and straightforward classification. It is fair to say that an entirely satisfactory subclassification of melanoma has not been achieved; some authorities have therefore stressed that melanoma should be considered as one entity and have discouraged the use of subtypes (Ackerman 1980, 1982; Ackerman and David 1986).

In the present chapter, we shall largely confine our discussion to those histological features which are most important for the differential diagnosis between melanoma and naevus, and only discuss melanoma subtypes in the context of this differential diagnosis. We feel that, even if the subclassification of melanoma as a whole is somewhat unsatisfactory, it is helpful to know of some of the different subtypes since this helps in differentiating melanomas from benign melanocytic lesions.

The differential diagnosis of melanoma versus naevus is at times exceedingly difficult. Cutaneous melanoma is a highly malignant tumour but, since most cases are discovered when they are still very small (when compared to malignant tumours of most internal organs), many patients are cured after primary treatment. Complete follow-up data of large numbers of cases are therefore needed in order to provide a satisfactory corroboration of histological features thought to differentiate between benign lesions (naevi) and malignant ones with a favourable prognosis (thin melanomas). Failure to appreciate this point may result in a spurious impression that the criteria proposed in a particular series of cases have been established beyond doubt, and that they can be safely relied on in diagnostic practice.

Furthermore, it should be borne in mind that, when a histological feature is used as an indicator of malignancy, its specificity should be extremely high, in view of the very large difference in prevalence between cutaneous naevi and melanoma; the predictive value of a diagnostic criterion is dependent on the relative prevalence of the entities requiring differentiation (Vecchio 1966).

Because of these reasons, as well as the marked variability of histological features encountered in cutaneous naevi, and in view of the fact that some entities have been described only relatively recently and may still be controversial, the differential diagnosis "naevus or melanoma" is not a straightforward and easy one.

Clinical Data

Site of the lesion, and sex and, most importantly, age of patient are significant parameters, and it is advisable not to report on pigmented lesions of the skin in the absence of this information (McGovern et al. 1986).

Diagnostic Specimen

In the large majority of cases, an excisional biopsy with narrow margins constitutes the proper type of biopsy. Punch biopsies or incisional biopsies are justified only in a small minority of instances (e.g. when the lesion is very small so that it is removed in its entirety by a punch biopsy, or when it is very large, or when the localization is awkward). The specimen should be fixed whole, transected and totally embedded, unless it is very large; in such instances, the thickest part, ulcerated parts, areas with different macroscopical appearances, and the site where the excisional margin is narrowest should always be included in the blocks taken. We discourage frozen section diagnosis of these lesions, since the morphology is suboptimal, step sections are generally not available, a relatively large amount of tissue is lost, and thickness measurements are not reliable (Nield et al. 1988).

Histological Features

Both architectural and cytological features are of importance in the diagnosis of melanoma. Much emphasis has been placed on the overall architecture ("silhouette") of the tumour (Ackerman 1980, 1989). Small, well-demarcated and (more or less) symmetrical melanocytic tumours are almost always benign; large, ill-defined and irregular melanocytic tumours are often malignant. Ascent and especially (pagetoid) lateral migration of tumour cells within the epidermis often indicates malignancy, and should be evaluated in conjunction with the above. Exceptions to these rules do occur, and will be briefly discussed in the subsequent sections.

Size

Most benign melanocytic tumours are smaller than 6 mm, and the large majority are under 1 cm in diameter. Congenital naevi, Spitz naevi, blue naevi, combined naevi, naevi of volar skin and dysplastic naevi are the most common benign naevus types which may exceed that size. At the time of diagnosis, melanomas are often larger than 1 cm in diameter, but obviously they may be smaller.

Lateral Demarcation

Most benign melanocytic lesions are well demarcated, indicating that their extreme lateral margin consists of melanocytic nests rather than a gradual petering-out of solitary cells. Moreover, the junctional lateral borders of benign lesions usually have a similar appearance at both sides; it is uncommon to see a sharp demarcation consisting of a melanocytic nest at one side, and a petering-out of single cells at the other. However, exceptions do occur: some Spitz naevi, pigmented spindle-cell naevi and dysplastic naevi may exhibit the above local variations in type of lateral spread.

Many melanomas have a poorly demarcated junctional lateral component, which may exhibit pagetoid spread of melanocytes (see blow), which is a stronger indicator of malignancy (Fig. 6.1). Exceptions include nodular melanomas (see below), which do not extend significantly at the lateral junctional borders.

Asymmetry

Benign melanocytic lesions are usually (more or less) symmetrical; in contrast, melanomas are often asymmetrical; the asymmetry may pertain to the lateral extension, extent of dermal involvement, architecture of epidermal and dermal component (nests, strands, nodules, sheets, fascicles), cell type, distribution and degree of pigmentation and host response.

Ascent of Atypical Melanocytes

In contrast to the large majority of benign melanocytic lesions, in which intraepidermal melanocytes retain their position at the dermoepidermal junction, melanoma cells are often seen to travel through the entire thickness of the epidermis (Fig. 6.2). This so-called melanocytic ascent may extend at the

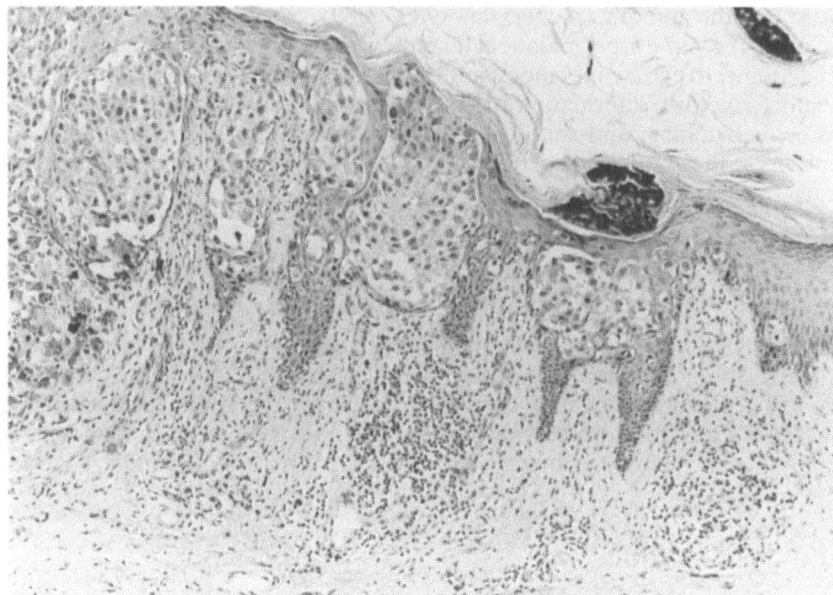

Fig. 6.1.   Irregular intraepidermal lateral spread of melanoma cells. Irregular nests as well as single cells are seen at the dermoepidermal junction and above it. H&E, × 90.

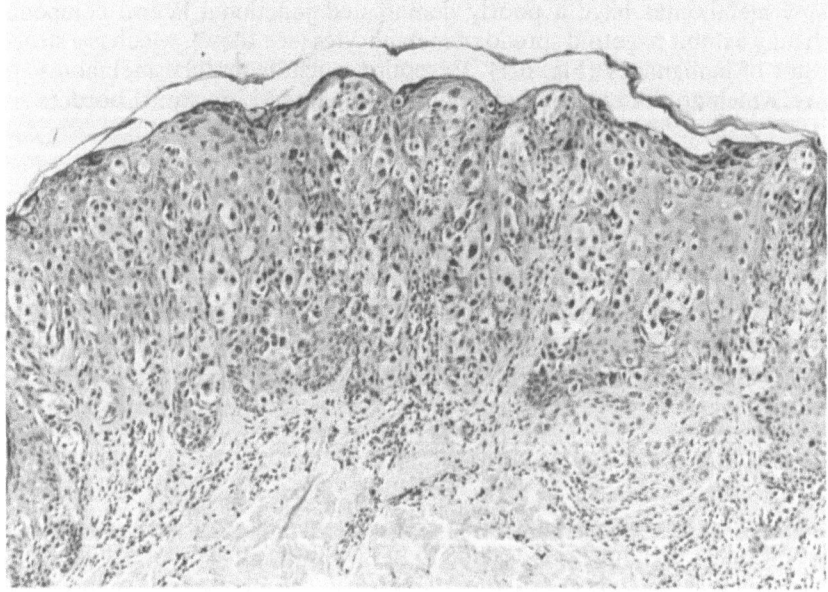

Fig. 6.2.   Ascent of melanoma cells throughout the entire thickness of the epidermis. H&E, × 90.

lateral borders of the tumour, resulting in pagetoid spread ("pagetoid" indicating that the histological picture mimics mammary and extramammary Paget's disease).

Ascent of melanocytes should not be confused with transepidermal elimination of melanocytic nests, which travel as large clumps through the epidermis to reach the surface. This phenomenon may be encountered in a large variety of benign melanocytic lesions, especially when large junctional melanocytic nests are formed.

Melanocytic ascent is absent in a minority of melanomas and, importantly, may be present in some benign lesions, albeit often to a lesser extent, and centrally rather than peripherally in the lesion. These benign lesions include Spitz naevus, pigmented spindle cell naevus, junctional naevus of volar skin, congenital naevus in early infancy, and, rarely, recurrent naevus. Apart from Paget's disease, some other non-melanocytic lesions may simulate melanocytic ascent: these include epidermotropic mycosis fungoides (Woringer Kolopp disease), histiocytosis X, pigmented Bowen's disease, some viral dermatoses, Toker's clear cells of the nipple, and clear cell paulosis of the skin. Usually, these alternatives are easily ruled out by the clinical data and appropriate histochemical and immune stains.

Pagetoid lateral spread of melanocytes is virtually diagnostic of melanoma: only rarely is it encountered in naevi recurring after incomplete removal, and in congenital naevi in infancy (especially in so-called satellite naevi associated with giant congenital naevi).

Intradermal Growth Pattern

In contrast to benign naevi, which generally exhibit a regular appearance of the intradermal component, often forming nests in the subepidermal zone and containing diffuse sheets and ill-defined fascicles in deeper parts and that are associated with a smaller and/or oval or elongated cell type, most melanomas show significant differences in cell type and tissue architecture between different areas of the tumour. Compact nodules may alternate with diffuse sheets of tumour cells or with cells scattered singly amidst a fibrotic stroma containing inflammatory cells.

Many melanomas do not exhibit "maturation" (transitions to a smaller and fusiform cell type towards the base of the tumour). However, exceptions are not uncommon; deep parts of melanomas may contain irregular and densely cellular areas with a small cell type. The large size and irregular shape of these aggregates, together with the presence of melanin and mitoses and, at high power, nuclear atypia indicate that such areas are an integral part of the malignant tumour rather than remnants of a pre-existent naevus. Rarely, the entire melanoma consists of such small "naevus-like" cells.

Epidermal and Dermal Reactive Changes

In melanomas, the epidermis often shows some reactive hyperplasia; however, this may be lacking, most commonly in lentigo maligna melanoma, which arises in chronically sun-damaged skin of elderly persons. Epidermal hyperplasia is not a very helpful diagnostic feature, since it is not uncommon in benign melanocytic lesions, and is a frequent finding in some, such as Spitz naevi.

Invasive melanoma often elicits an inflammatory antitumour response, which most characteristically takes the shape of a band-like, predominantly lymphocytic infiltrate, located at the base of the tumour. There is often accompanying fibrosis and angiogenesis. Characteristically, these reactive features may vary from place to place, in extent as well as in quality (some areas containing an inflammatory infiltrate, others showing fibrosis), adding to the asymmetrical and irregular architecture of the tumour.

Melanoma

Below, brief mention will be made of the four main subtypes of melanoma, as well as a number of less-common melanoma subtypes that are associated with specific diagnostic or therapeutic problems.

Mainly based on the work of Clark et al. (1969), the large majority of cutaneous melanomas are classified as superficial spreading, nodular, lentigo maligna and acral lentiginous melanoma. This subclassification is based mainly on the pattern of spread of the intraepidermal tumour component and, in the case of acral lentiginous melanoma (Reed 1976), also on localization.

Superficial Spreading Melanoma

Superficial spreading melanoma is the most common subtype, comprising about two-thirds of cases. The distinguishing feature is the presence of pagetoid spread of tumour cells within the epidermis over a distance of at least three rete ridges lateral to the lateral border of the intradermal tumour component (Fig. 6.1). In most instances the tumour cells are epithelioid in type, but they may be oval and dendritic, and in some instances this is associated with a lentiginous type of growth, along the epidermal basement membrane rather than a pagetoid type (at all levels of the epidermis).

Nodular Melanoma

Nodular melanoma lacks significant intraepidermal spread of tumour cells within the epidermis lateral to the intradermal tumour component. It will be obvious that a superficial spreading melanoma will change to a nodular melanoma once the intradermal component outgrows the intraepidermal part. Some nodular melanomas have a short clinical history, and exhibit an exophytic growth pattern. Such tumours, which are often thick and ulcerated and which are accordingly associated with a poor prognosis, have sometimes been referred to as "*polypoid melanomas*" (Fig. 6.3).

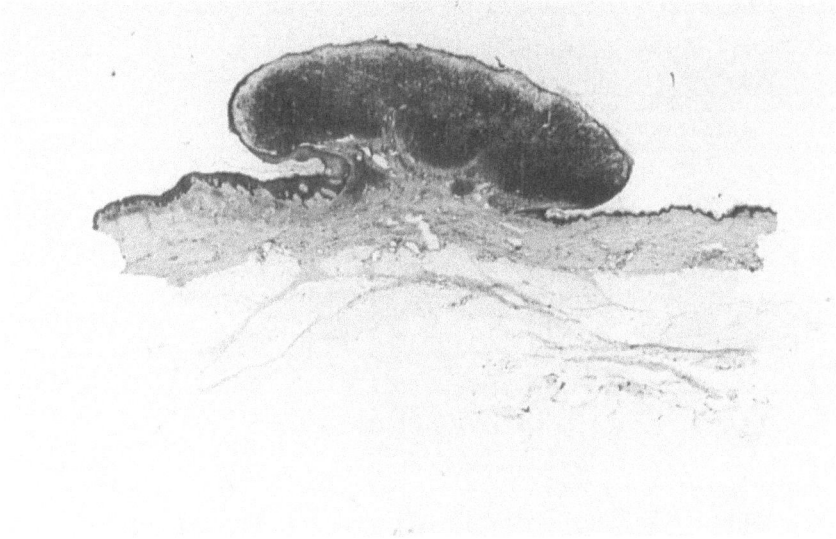

Fig. 6.3. "Polypoid melanoma". The entire tumour is raised above the original level of the epidermis. H&E, × 4.

Lentigo Maligna Melanoma

Lentigo maligna melanoma arises on the basis of an often long-standing flat irregular pigmentation of sun-damaged skin in elderly patients, which histologically corresponds to a proliferation of pigmented dendritic melanocytes, usually in a lentiginous arrangement with or without nests, and exhibiting varying degrees of nuclear atypia, within an atrophic epidermis (lentigo maligna, morbus Dubreuilh, Hutchinson's melanotic freckle). Lentigo maligna melanomas may exhibit a wide spectrum of histological appearances, ranging from diffusely growing spindle-cell melanomas to nodular, epithelioid cell-type melanomas (Fig. 6.4). Despite early claims to the contrary, the prognosis of this melanoma subtype is similar to that of other subtypes, when stratified for major histological prognostic indicators such as thickness and the presence of ulceration (Koh et al. 1984).

Acral Lentiginous Melanoma

Acral lentiginous melanoma (Reed 1976) occurs on volar (palmar and plantar) skin, whereas melanomas of juxtacutaneous mucous membranes often show a similar histology. The intraepidermal component of these melanomas usually consists of dendritic atypical melanocytes which grow preferentially along the epidermal basement membrane, as solitary units, and this is often associated with some degree of epidermal hyperplasia. *Subungual melanomas* also belong to this category. These tumours are often associated with a significant delay by both patient and doctor, so that at the time of their removal they have often deeply penetrated underlying tissues, which is associated with a poor prognosis.

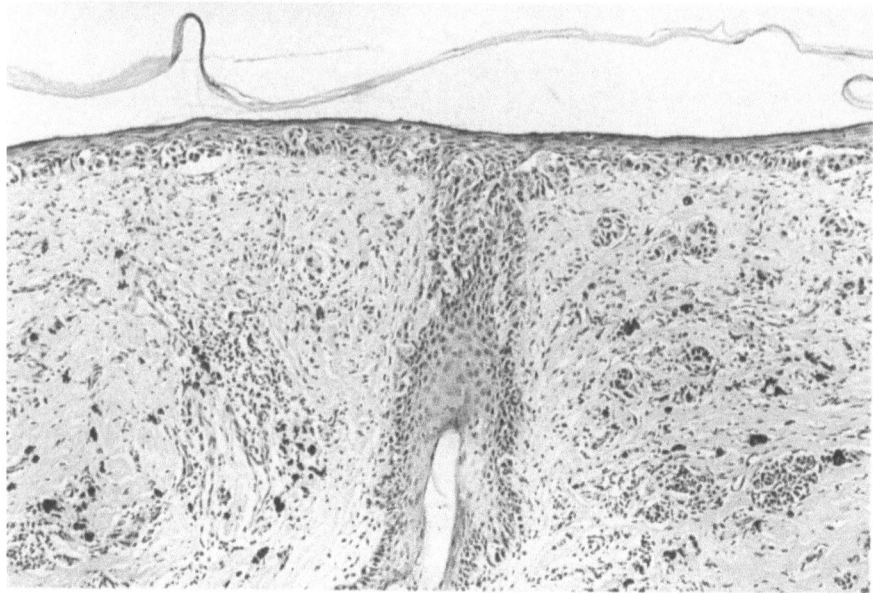

Fig. 6.4. Lentigo maligna melanoma. The dermoepidermal junction contains an almost continuous proliferation of atypical melanocytes, some of which ascend into the upper layers of the atrophic epidermis. Small nests of tumour cells deeply penetrate the dermis. H&E, × 35.

Some additional melanoma subtypes, which are not necessarily mutually exclusive with the above main subtypes, warrant a brief separate discussion in view of the specific diagnostic and therapeutic problems with which they are associated.

Desmoplastic Melanoma

Desmoplastic melanoma often arises in sun-exposed skin, most commonly in the head and neck region, in later adult life with a male preponderance. Clinically, a flat and irregular pigmentation indicative of lentigo maligna may be present, but in its absence, the cutaneous nodule is devoid of clinical tell-tale signs of malignancy or a melanocytic nature. Excision of such a lesion is often performed under a provisional clinical diagnosis of a non-neoplastic or benign lesion. Delay by patient and doctor together with initial inadequate treatment results in a relatively poor prognosis, related to a high local recurrence rate (Egbert et al. 1988; Jain and Allen 1989). Local recurrence is particularly ominous in the *neurotropic type* of desmoplastic melanoma, where preferential perineural growth of tumour cells results in macroscopically visible thickening of nerves. Histologically, the tumour consists of a diffuse proliferation of elongated melanocytes, which are often wholly amelanocytic and therefore may not be recognized as such. Between the tumour cells, a varying amount of newly formed collagen is present (Fig. 6.5). The tumour cells have greatly elongated nuclei, which have pointed ends; nuclear chromatin is moderately dense. Intranuclear cytoplasmic pseudoinclusions, S-100 positivity, the presence of traces of melanin

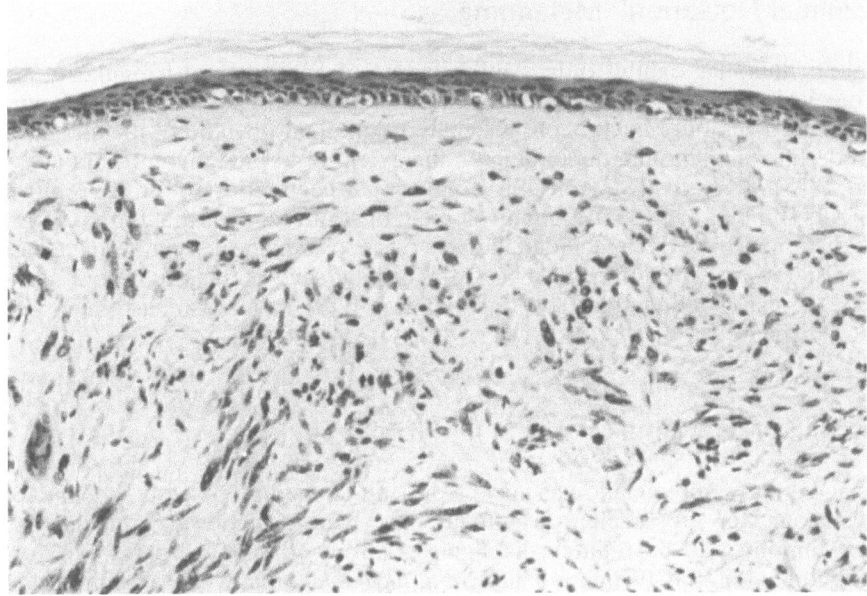

Fig. 6.5. Desmoplastic melanoma. A diffuse proliferation of atypical elongated tumour cells is present in the dermis. Note epidermal atrophy and the presence of slightly atypical melanocytes at the dermoepidermal junction. H&E, × 185.

and the ultrastructural features (very similar to those of Schwann cells) suggest the correct diagnosis.

Verrucous Naevoid Melanoma

This melanoma type shows a close architectural resemblance to the common benign papillomatous compound naevus (Suster et al. 1987). It is usually much larger, the number of junctional melanocytes often greatly exceeds that in papillomatous naevi, mitoses are usually found in the dermal component (but may be scarce) and there may be small microsatellites in the vicinity. When one seriously considers the possibility of melanoma, these tumours are not easily misdiagnosed as naevi; the danger is, that these melanomas are dismissed as benign because of their deceptive low-power papillomatous appearance.

Malignant Blue Naevus

The differential diagnosis between cellular blue naevus and malignant blue naevus is very difficult. It is useful to bear in mind that malignant blue naevus is exceedingly rare and usually shows a brisk mitotic activity as well as an early tendency for necrosis (Goldenhersh et al. 1988; Temple-Camp et al. 1988). Benign cellular blue naevi may be several centimetres in size, may exhibit a pushing growth pattern, especially upon reaching the subcutaneous fatty tissue, may contain mitoses, and lack "maturation". One should therefore guard against over-diagnosis of cellular blue naevi as malignant blue naevi.

"Minimal Deviation" Melanoma

Some melanomas exhibit only a mild degree of architectural irregularity and cytological atypia, and are therefore more difficult to distinguish from benign naevi. Such tumours have been designated "minimal deviation" melanoma or "borderline" melanoma, depending on the extent of dermal involvement (Reed et al. 1975). A relatively favourable prognosis has been reported for this group of tumours (Phillips et al. 1986), but an element of doubt remains that perhaps some benign lesions have been included in the series upon which such claims have been based in view of the difficulties of distinguishing such melanomas from naevi. Also, the exact delineation from the common types of melanoma remains less than satisfactory.

Spitz-like Melanoma

We agree that some melanomas may be difficult to distinguish from benign naevi but, in our view, insufficient arguments have been provided to conclude that these tumours can be reliably distinguished from other melanomas. The one exception to this may be the so-called *Spitz-like melanoma*, which exhibits a close resemblance to Spitz naevus, but which is usually larger, may be ulcerated, exhibits pagetoid lateral spread of tumour cells as well as confluent junctional activity; whereas at the base there is lack of maturation, a compact pushing pattern of growth, and mitoses, which may be numerous and may include atypical ones. Such tumours have been claimed to give rise to small regional lymph node deposits but not to distant metastases (Smith et al. 1989). However, a case recently encountered by us gave rise to massive lymph node involvement after a short period of time.

Melanoma in Childhood

Childhood melanoma is very rare, but has been reported even in neonates. A significant proportion of melanomas in childhood occur in the context of congenital naevi, and some others are associated with xeroderma pigmentosum or the familial dysplastic naevus syndrome; therefore, one should be very conservative with the diagnosis of childhood melanoma outside these settings. The histological features of melanoma in childhood are similar to those occurring later in life except for part of the early childhood melanomas occurring in giant congenital naevi; such tumours often arise deep within the naevus and show a very varied spectrum of appearances (Hendrickson and Ross 1981).

Since Spitz naevus and its variants are more prevalent in childhood, and since common acquired naevi may show a more conspicuous junctional component, one should guard against over-diagnosis of melanoma in this age group. The prognosis of childhood melanoma appears to be similar to that in adulthood, when stratified for the main prognostic parameters such as thickness, site and the presence of ulceration (Roth et al. 1990).

Cutaneous Metastasis Versus (Second) Primary Melanoma

The differentiation between a cutaneous metastasis of melanoma and a second primary tumour is of prognostic significance. In the latter instance, the prognosis is comparable to that of the thickest of the two primary melanomas, disregarding the other one, whereas in the case of cutaneous metastases, the context is that of (locoregional or even distant) metastatic disease.

In the large majority of cases, the distinction can be made with confidence on histological grounds. Most cutaneous metastases are confined to the dermis, whereas the large majority of primary melanomas have an intraepidermal component. Some metastases, however, also involve the epidermis ("epidermotropic" melanoma metastases, Kornberg et al. 1978). In such cases the lateral extension of the dermal component generally exceeds that of the epidermal one. Ascent of tumour cells is rare, and the epidermis is often thinned rather than hyperplastic. An epidermal collarette may be formed at either side, intravascular tumour cells are relatively commonly seen, and, importantly, the overall appearance is rather bland. The tumour cells exhibit less variation than in most primary melanomas, whereas reactive inflammation and fibrosis are absent or mild and do not show the variations seen in most primary tumours (Fig. 6.6).

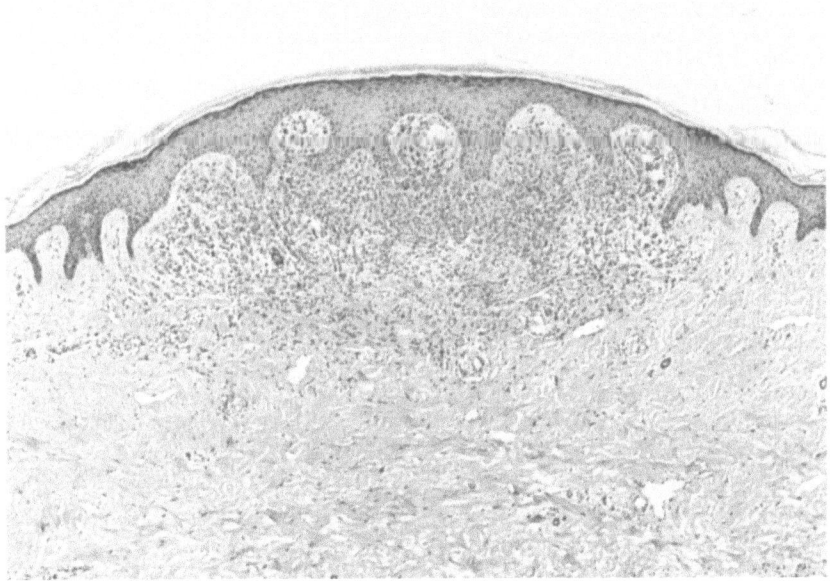

Fig. 6.6. Cutaneous melanoma metastasis. In this instance, the overlying epidermis is uninvolved; note also the absence of an inflammatory response as well as the relatively bland appearance of the lesion. H&E, × 35.

Prognosis of Melanoma

A very large number of prognostic factors have been identified in melanoma. In routine diagnostic practice, it is wise to use a fixed set of well-corroborated prognostic factors. Tumour stage, site, maximal thickness as assessed histologically (Breslow 1970, 1980), level of cutaneous invasion (Clark et al. 1969), the presence of ulceration and microsatellitosis are the most important of these.

Routine Diagnostic Pathology Report of Melanoma

A report should include the diagnosis of melanoma and a statement concerning the completeness of resection, as well as an assessment of the main prognostic parameters mentioned above. The choice of the clinically free margin to be resected, as well as the likelihood of locoregional or distant tumour recurrence, depend greatly on these factors.

References

Ackerman AB (1980) Malignant melanoma, a unifying concept. Hum Pathol 11:591–595

Ackerman AB (1982) Disagreements with the current classification of malignant melanomas. Am J Surg Pathol 6:733–743

Ackerman AB (1989) Differentiation of benign from malignant neoplasms by silhouette. Am J Dermatopathol 11:297–300

Ackerman AB, David KM (1986) A unifying concept of malignant melanoma: biologic aspects. Hum Pathol 17:438–440

Breslow A (1970) Thickness, cross-sectional area and depth of invasion in the prognosis of cutaneous melanoma. Ann Surg 172:902–908

Breslow A (1980) Prognosis in cutaneous melanoma: tumor thickness as a guide to treatment. Pathol Ann 15–I:1–22

Clark WH, From L, Bernardino E, Mihm MC (1969) The histogenesis and biologic behavior of primary human malignant melanomas of the skin. Cancer Res 29:705–726

Egbert B, Kempson R, Sagebiel R (1988) Desmoplastic malignant melanoma. A clinicohistopathologic study of 25 cases. Cancer 62:2033–2041

Goldenhersh MA, Sarin RC, Barnill RL, Stenn KS (1988) Malignant blue nevus. Case report and literature review. J Am Acad Dermatol 19:712–722

Hendrickson MR, Ross JC (1981) Neoplasms arising in congenital giant naevi. Morphologic study of seven cases and a review of the literature. Am J Surg Pathol 5:109–135

Jain S, Allen PW (1989) Desmoplastic malignant melanoma and its variants. A study of 45 cases. Am J Surg Pathol 13:358–373

Koh H, Michalik E, Sober AJ et al. (1984) Lentigo maligna melanoma has no better prognosis than other types of melanoma. J Clin Oncol 2:994–1001

Kornberg R, Harris M, Ackerman AB (1978) Epidermotropically metastatic malignant melanoma. Arch Dermatol 114:67–69

McGovern VJ, Cochran AJ, Van der Esch EP, Little JH, MacLennan R (1986) The classification of malignant melanoma, its histological reporting and registration: a revision of the 1972 Sydney classification. Pathology 18:12–21

Nield DV, Saad MN, Khoo CTK, Lott M, Ali MH (1988) Tumour thickness in malignant melanoma: the limitation of frozen section. Br J Plast Surg 41:403–407

Phillips ME, Margolis RJ, Merot Y, Sober AJ, Reed RJ, Muhlbauer JE, Mihm MC (1986) The spectrum of minimal deviation melanoma: a clinicopathologic study of 21 cases. Hum Pathol 17:796–806

Reed RJ (1976) Acral lentiginous melanoma. In: New concepts in surgical pathology of the skin, Wiley, New York, pp 87–97

Reed R RJ, Ichinose H, Clark WH, Mihm JC (1975) Common and uncommon melanocytic nevi and borderline melanomas. Semin Oncol 2:119–147

Roth ME, Grant-Kels JM, Kuhn K, Greenberg RD, Hurwitz S (1990) Melanoma in children. J Am Acad Dermatol 22:265–274

Smith KJ, Skelton HG, Lupton GP, Graham JH (1989) Spindle and epithelioid cell nevi with atypia and metastasis (malignant Spitz nevus). Am J Surg Pathol 13:931–939

Suster S, Ronnen M, Bubis JJ (1987) Verrucous pseudonevoid melanoma. J Surg Oncol 36:134–137

Temple-Camp CRE, Saxe N, King H (1988) Benign and malignant cellular blue nevus. A clinocopathologic study of 30 cases. Am J Dermatopathol 10:289–296

Vecchio TJ (1966) Predictive value of a single diagnostic test in unselected populations. N Engl J Med 274:1171–1173

7   Histopathological Differential Diagnosis

N. P. Smith

The diagnosis of any cutaneous lesion is based on clinical and histopathological criteria. Neither of these sets of criteria are infallible and indeed in histopathological diagnosis of melanocytic lesions different criteria assume varying degrees of importance, depending on the setting in which they are found. The diagnosis of malignant melanoma has important implications for the patient. Studies on the results of various treatment protocols for malignant melanoma and data on long-term survival are obviously invalid if the original diagnosis is not correct.

There are many clinical lesions that may on occasions simulate malignant melanoma and the clinician's suspicions are normally aroused by the presence of a lesion which is heavily pigmented. Many of the lesions mistaken clinically for malignant melanoma are malformations or tumours of blood vessels, or contain haemosiderin pigment. Fortunately, these lesions do not normally pose a problem for the diagnostic histopathologist. Examples of such conditions include haemangioma, haemosiderotic histiocytoma, venous lakes, pyogenic granuloma, Kaposi's sarcoma and haemosiderin deposition as a result of trauma (e.g. talon noir and nail bed haemorrhage after trauma).

On occasion other non-vascular or non-haemosiderin containing dermal tumours, especially if they are pigmented, may cause clinical confusion. Examples include apocrine cystadenoma and eccrine spiradenoma. Again, there is normally no problem differentiating such lesions from malignant melanoma histologically, although some histiocytomas, especially the recently described epithelioid histiocytoma, may closely mimic a melanocytic tumour (Wilson Jones et al. 1989).

Melanin itself causes pigmentation in a wide variety of lesions. Some of these are epidermal lesions, such as seborrhoeic warts, melanoacanthoma (Mishima and Pinkus 1960), and pigmented Bowen's disease and Bowenoid papulosis. The presence of exogenous pigment deposited in the dermis, such as occurs in tattoos, may sometimes simulate a melanocytic lesion but normally the histological picture is characteristic. One situation where intradermal foreign pigment may produce a histological picture with a superficial resemblance to a melanocytic lesion occurs when Monsel's solution is used as a haemostatic agent following curettage or cutaneous surgery (Amazon et al. 1980; Olmstead et al. 1980; Wood and Severin 1980). Monsel's solution is a solution of ferric subsulphate and in some patients following application of this agent to a wound there develops, over a period of time, extensive permeation of the substance throughout the dermal connective tissue. The solution is taken up by macrophages and also coats collagen bundles. Commonly, irregularly shaped clumps of refractile dark-brown and bluish-black material are present in the dermis and a foreign body giant cell reaction is also often seen (Figs 7.1 and 7.2). The presence of refractile aggregations of pigment, the confirmation that this material is positive with a Perls' stain and the lack of any obvious cytological atypia or mitoses helps to differentiate this unusual lesion from a melanocytic neoplasm.

Another skin disorder that can histologically closely mimic a superficial or intraepidermal malignant melanoma is that of cutaneous T-cell lymphoma. Epidermotropic mycosis fungoides or other forms of cutaneous T-cell lymphoma, such as Pagetoid reticulosis, may reveal atypical hyperchromatic mononuclear cells within the epidermis and forming nests near the epidermodermal junction. Many of the atypical cells within the epidermis have a clear halo and can closely simulate atypical melanocytes leading to an erroneous diagnosis (Fig. 7.3). Features that aid a differentiation of epidermotropic T-cell lymphoma from malignant melanoma in situ include the following:

1. The absence of truly expansile nests of tumour cells at the epidermodermal junction, most of the atypical cells lying within the epidermis

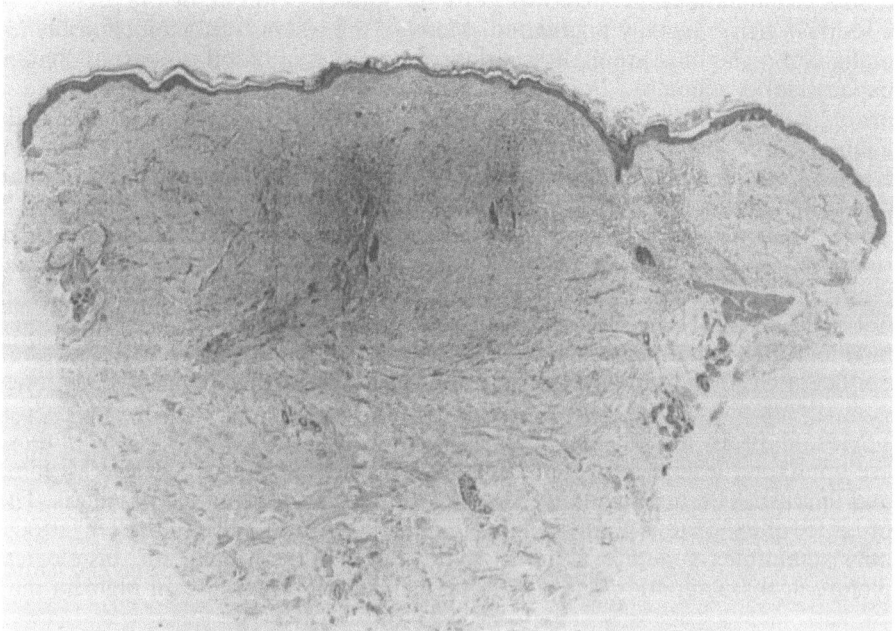

Fig. 7.1. Low power view of lesion treated with Monsel's solution following surgery. Extensive fibrosis and patchy pigmentation are seen.

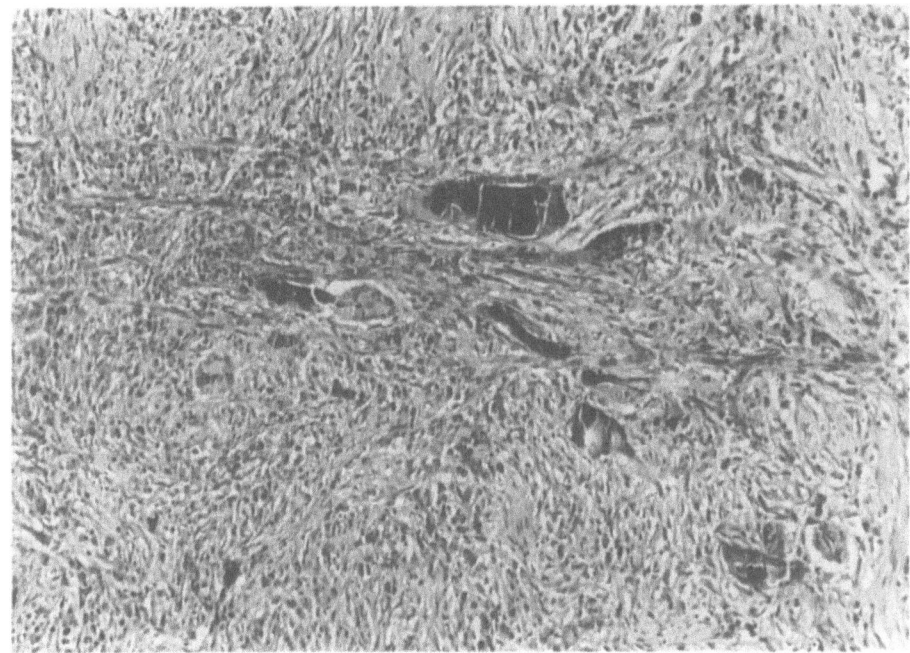

Fig. 7.2. High power view from the same case as Fig. 7.1. Fibrosis of connective tissue, pigment-containing macrophages and irregular refractile deposits of pigment.

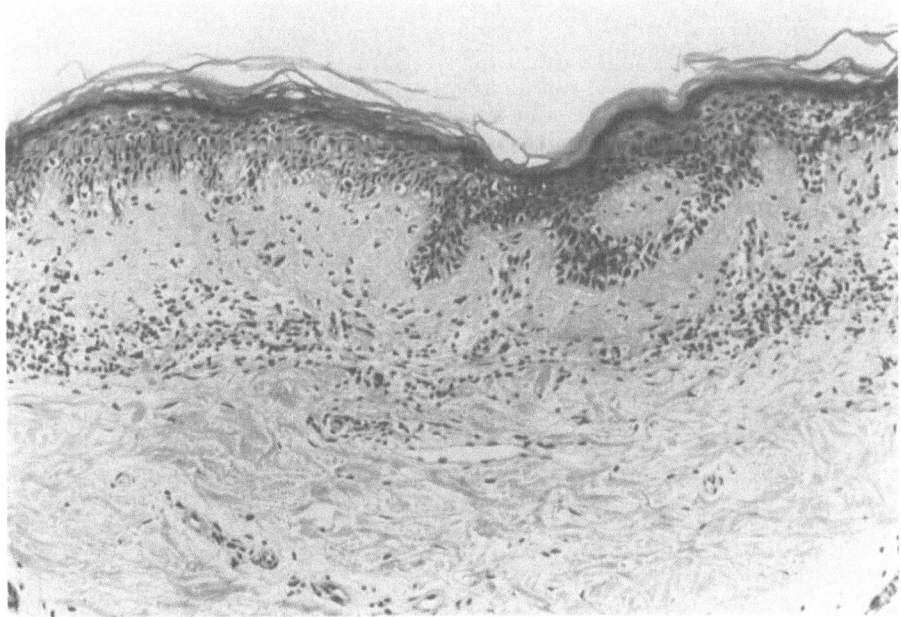

Fig. 7.3. Hyperchromatic mononuclear cells at the epidermodermal junction and within the epidermis simulating a melanocytic lesion in a case of cutaneous T-cell lymphoma.

2. The presence of atypical mononuclear cells within the dermal infiltrate, although in cases where the dermal infiltrate is sparse these may be hard to find.

3. Psoriasiform hyperplasia of the epidermis is often present in Pagetoid reticulosis.

4. Immunohistochemistry is most helpful in confirming the lymphocytic nature of the cells within the dermis and colonizing the epidermis (Fig. 7.4). It should be noted, however, that in epidermotropic cutaneous T-cell lymphoma the intraepidermal mononuclear cells often lose some of their pan T-cell antigens. This feature has been termed "discordance of antigen expression" (Michie et al. 1990).

The clinical features of most forms of cutaneous T-cell lymphoma rarely suggest malignant melanoma but in the absence of helpful clinical information, the diagnostic pathologist may find accurate interpretation of these lesions difficult.

Skin disorders other than cutaneous T-cell lymphoma where histologically there is colonization of the epidermis by atypical keratinocytes or other cells can sometimes produce a picture of pagetoid or superficial spreading melanoma. The most important of these conditions are Paget's disease itself and the various disorders that show the Borst–Jadassohn phenomenon, including intraepidermal squamous cell carcinoma and Bowen's disease and some forms of eccrine porocarcinoma. The shape, size and nature of the intraepidermal nests of tumour

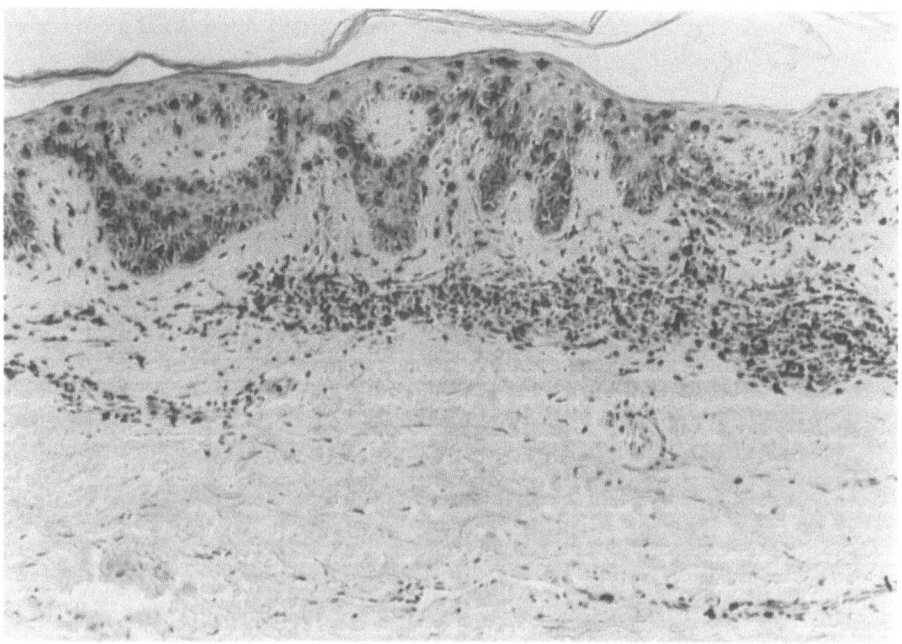

Fig. 7.4. Labelling with leukocyte common antigen confirms the lymphocytic nature of the cells both in the dermis and epidermis in the same case of cutaneous T-cell lymphoma illustrated in Fig. 7.3.

cells however in these conditions can usually be differentiated from the large pagetoid epithelioid cells seen in malignant melanoma of the superficial spreading type.

There are many different melanocytic lesions that can cause diagnostic problems for the histopathologist. Based on the experience with consultation material received by the author at the Department of Histopathology in the St John's Dermatology Centre, it seems that lesions that cause diagnostic confusion can be classified into three groups: (1) benign melanocytic lesions that have some histological characteristics normally associated with malignant melanoma; (2) examples of genuine malignant melanoma that exhibit some histological features normally associated with benign naevi, and (3) superficial, predominantly junctional, melanocytic proliferations exhibiting some degree of cytological and architectural atypia; this group includes so-called dysplastic naevi and related lesions. In the rest of this chapter on the histopathological differential diagnosis of malignant melanoma I will concentrate on lesions coming under the headings of groups (1) and (3) above.

Benign Melanocytic Lesions with Histological Characteristics Normally Associated with Malignant Melanoma

Spitz Naevi (Juvenile Melanoma, Spindle and Epithelioid Cell Naevi) (Echevarria and Ackerman 1967; Coskey and Mehregan 1973; Paniago-Pereira et al. 1978; Gartmann and Ganser 1984)

Sophie Spitz (1948) in her seminal paper drew attention to a form of malignant melanoma occurring in prepubertal children with characteristic histological features which were different from common malignant melanoma occurring in adults and also different from ordinary childhood naevi. The course of these melanomas was noted to be benign. It is now realized that the lesion described by Spitz is a variant of benign cellular naevus. Although the lesions are more common in the younger age group, Spitz naevi can be found at all ages. The typical clinical appearance is that of a symmetrical, moderately firm, protuberant papular lesion occurring in a young patient. The lesions may occur in any site but are particularly common on the face. Usually the lesions are flesh-coloured or pinkish-red reflecting the vascularity which is so often seen histologically. There may be a history of fairly rapid growth which frequently brings the patient to the attention of the doctor. Multiple and grouped or agminate lesions of Spitz naevi have also been well described (Bourlond 1971; Brownstein 1972; Gould and Bleehen 1980; Lancer et al. 1983).

Histologically typical Spitz naevi are usually symmetrical and the cells in the deeper parts of the lesion are frequently small and more closely resemble ordinary naevus cells than the cells in the superficial part of the tumour (Fig. 7.5). The superficial tumour cells are frequently large with abundant cytoplasm, may have more than one nucleus and the nuclei may exhibit cytoplasmic inclusions

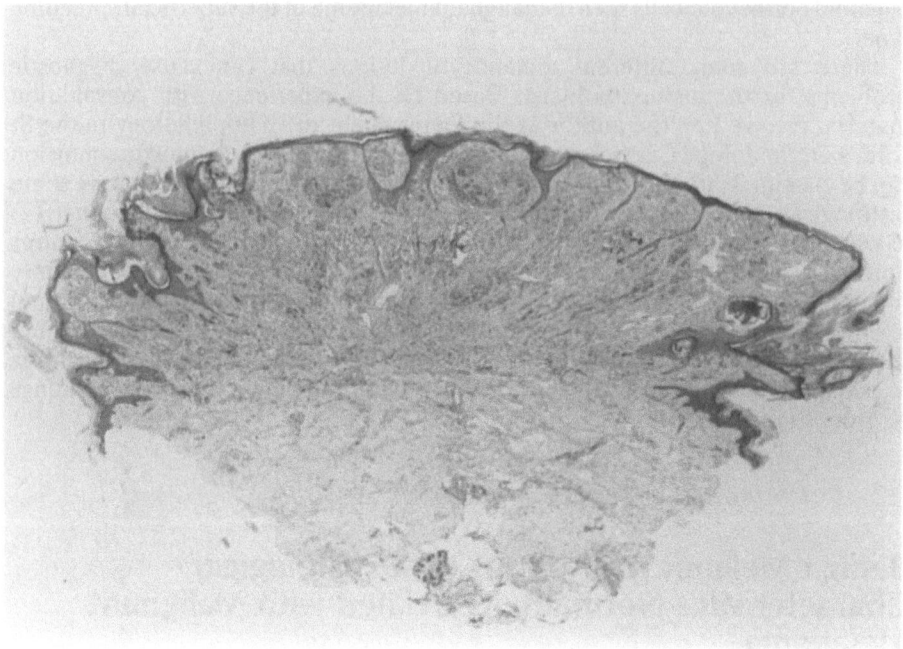

Fig. 7.5. Low power view of a Spitz naevus showing overall symmetry and a degree of epidermal hyperplasia.

(Fig. 7.6). Despite the sometimes marked cytological atypia of these cells, nuclear atypia and mitoses are much less common. The tendency of naevus cells in the deeper portion of a Spitz naevus to be smaller than the often bizarre cells in the superficial portions is sometimes referred to as maturation. The epidermis overlying a Spitz naevus is usually acanthotic and occasionally this acanthosis may amount to pseudoepitheliomatous hyperplasia. The junctional component in many Spitz naevi is not very prominent and serial sections may be needed to identify this. Intraepidermal spread of tumour cells is not normally seen in Spitz naevi and if this is a prominent feature malignant melanoma should be considered. Eosinophilic globules near the epidermodermal junction, known as Kamino bodies (Kamino et al. 1979), are commoner in Spitz naevi than in malignant melanoma but are certainly not specifically diagnostic (Liftin et al. 1985). The tumour cells of Spitz naevi are frequently non-pigmented and the growth pattern tends to be infiltrative rather than expansile with small groups and strands of tumour cells extending in between collagen bundles (Fig. 7.7). In malignant melanoma in its vertical growth phase there is normally evidence of expansile growth. The stroma of a Spitz naevus is often oedematous, particularly in the superficial portion and large numbers of dilated small blood vessels may also be seen.

Several histological variants of classical Spitz naevi have been described, the most important of which are the so-called desmoplastic naevus (Barr et al. 1980) where thin strands of naevus cells are embedded in a somewhat fibrotic stroma, these lesions on occasion giving rise to a mistaken diagnosis of desmoplastic

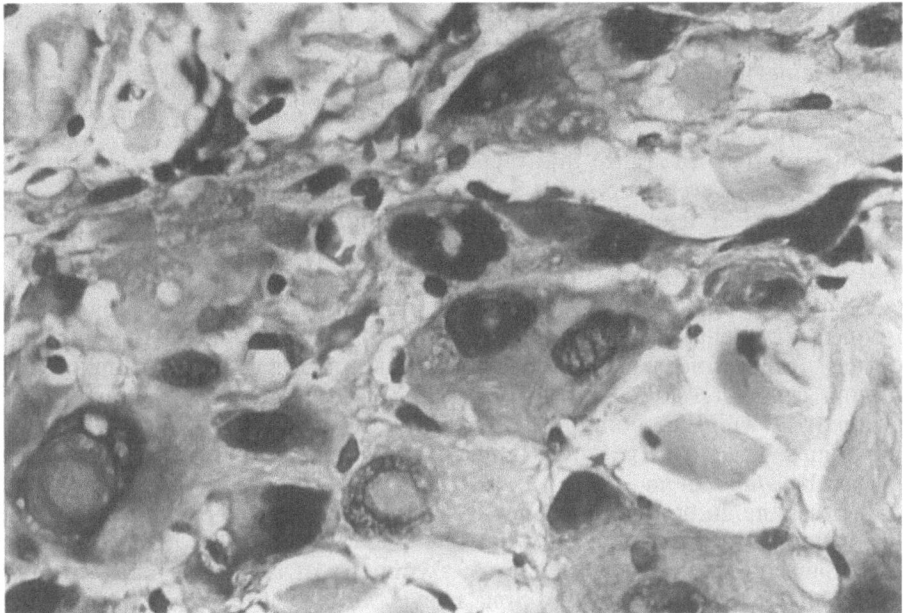

Fig. 7.6. Large bizarre multinucleate epithelioid cells from the superficial portion of a Spitz naevus. Note the presence of intranuclear cytoplasmic inclusions.

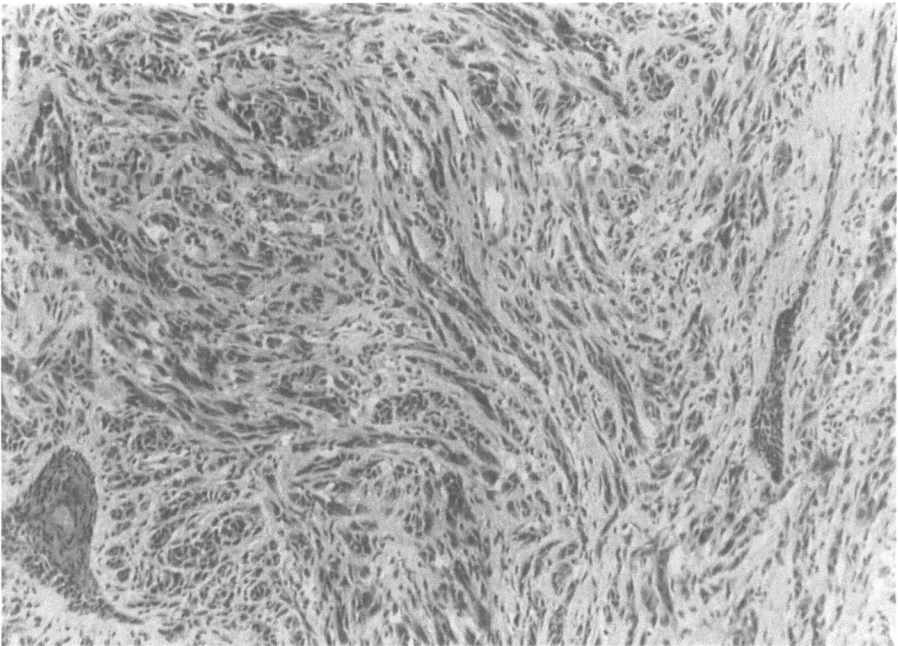

Fig. 7.7. The "raining down" pattern of epithelioid and spindle cells extending in between collagen bundles.

melanoma, and the combined naevus (Rogers et al. 1985) where elements of Spitz naevus are present together with elements elsewhere in the lesion of a conventional intradermal naevus or blue naevus. These combined naevi may give rise to concern because of the asymmetry of the lesion at low power microscopic examination.

It is important to realize that there is no single criterion that is absolute in allowing the differentiation of a Spitz naevus from malignant melanoma. The histopathological features of a typical Spitz tumour and a typical malignant melanoma are illustrated schematically in Figs. 7.8 and 7.9. The malignant melanoma shows low-power asymmetry with an expansile growth pattern, cytological atypia and mitotic figures at all levels of the lesion, pigment is frequently present and there may be a lymphocytic host response in the subjacent dermis. In pagetoid malignant melanoma intraepidermal spread of epithelioid tumour cells is an additional feature. The Spitz tumour on the other hand is symmetrical with the tumour cells showing maturation in the deeper portions of the lesions. The growth pattern is infiltrative rather than expansile and the stroma is vascular and oedematous.

In assessing an unusual melanocytic tumour the following features should at least suggest to the pathologist that one might be dealing with a malignant melanoma rather than a Spitz naevus: asymmetry of the lesion (apart from in examples of so-called combined Spitz naevi), an expansile growth pattern, the presence of intralesional transformation with groups of cells of quite different cytomorphology present next to each other with an abrupt transition from one cell type to the other, the presence of intraepidermal tumour cells, marked

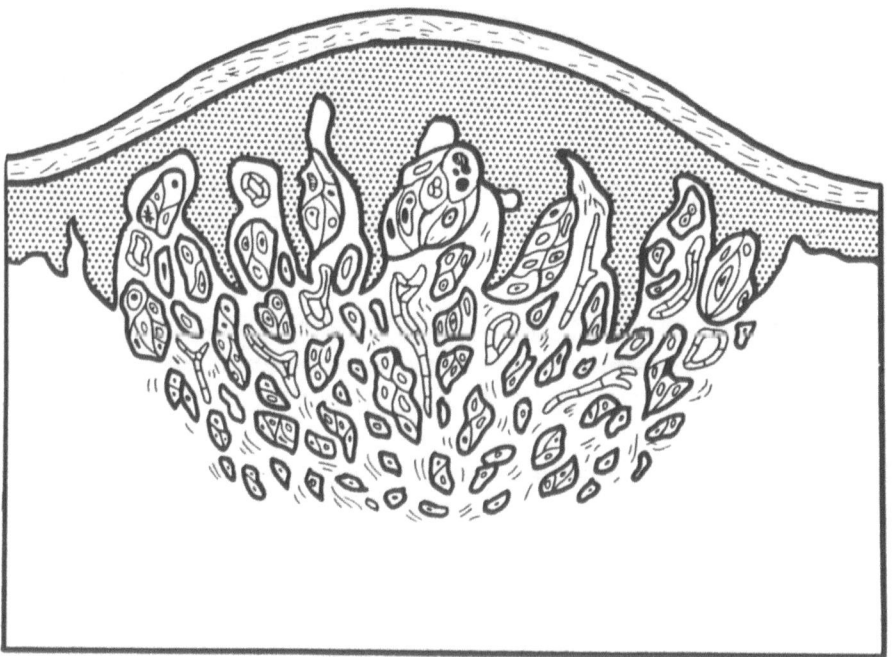

Fig. 7.8. Diagrammatic representation of the pathology of a typical Spitz naevus. Reproduced from Smith (1987), with permission.

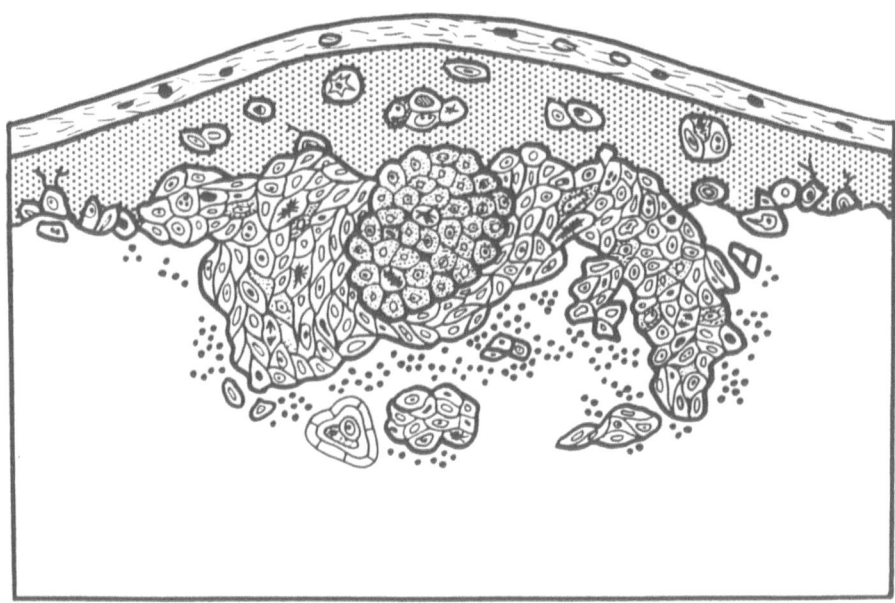

Fig. 7.9. Diagrammatic representation of the pathology of a typical superficial spreading malignant melanoma. Reproduced from Smith (1987), with permission.

nuclear atypia, and the presence of mitoses, particularly if these are numerous, atypical or found in the deeper portions of the lesion. As with all melanocytic tumours it is essential that the clinician provides good clinical details of the lesion if an accurate diagnosis is to be achieved.

Pigmented Spindle Cell Tumour (Pigmented Spindle Cell Naevus, Reed's Tumour) (Reed et al. 1975; Gartmann 1980; Sagebiel et al. 1984; Smith 1987; Barnhill and Mihm 1989)

Although this lesion is regarded by some as a variant of Spitz naevus, it has different clinical and histological characteristics. In common with a Spitz naevus the lesion is seen in children and young adults more frequently than in the elderly. Pigmented spindle cell tumours are twice as common in females as males and although they may occur on any area of the body, the lower limb is the site most frequently affected. Unlike most Spitz naevi, the lesions are very heavily pigmented, often suggesting to the clinician a diagnosis of malignant melanoma. The lesions are usually symmetrical with regular borders and rarely exceed 1 cm in size, often being much smaller.

   Histological examination of pigmented spindle cell tumours usually reveals a superficial symmetrical compound melanocytic tumour with sharp lateral demarcation and some degree of epidermal hyperplasia over the lesion (Fig. 7.10). Unlike many Spitz naevi, the junctional component is very prominent and in some cases is almost continuous. Although occasional intraepidermal tumour

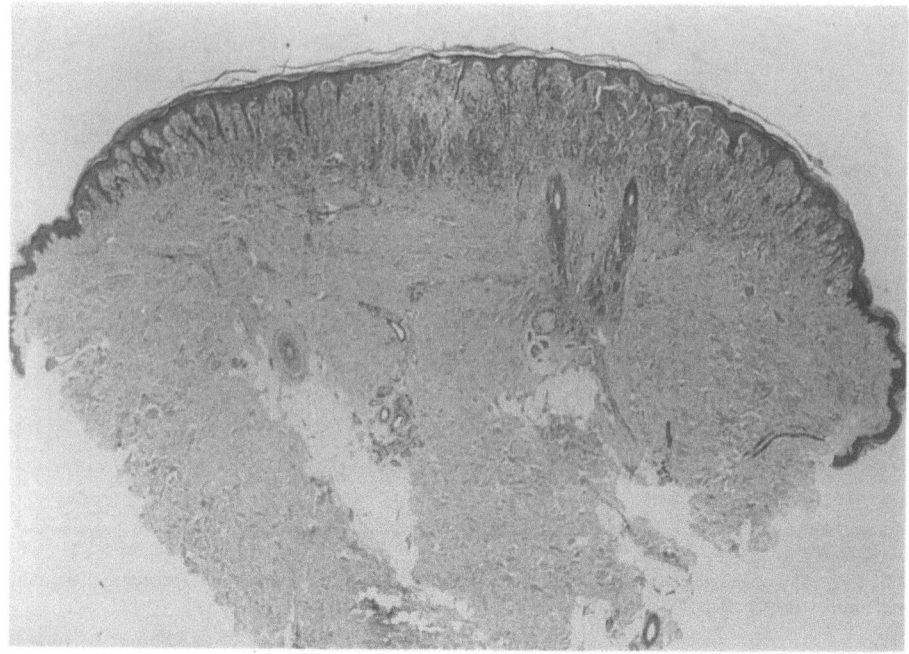

Fig. 7.10.   Low power view of a pigmented spindle cell tumour. Note the symmetry, superficiality of the lesion and the sharp lateral demarcation.

cells may be seen in this lesion, genuine pagetoid spread throughout all levels of the epidermis is most uncommon. the dermal component of the tumour is composed of medium to large size spindle cells, often with large nuclei and prominent nucleoli. The cytoplasm of these cells contains finely dispersed melanin pigment and pigmented macrophages are commonly seen within and around the tumour (Fig. 7.11). Mitoses may be seen in this lesion and occasionally abnormal mitoses are also found (Fig. 7.12). The pattern of growth, unlike that seen in Spitz naevi, is expansile with confluent nests of spindle cells appearing to "push down" into the underlying dermis. Below the tumour there is usually a chronic inflammatory cell infiltrate. Pigmented spindle cell naevi are important as they are frequently misdiagnosed both by clinicians and pathologists as malignant melanoma. Despite the increased number of publications in recent years on the subject the lesion is still under-recognized.

   The tumour can be distinguished histopathologically from Spitz naevi by its growth pattern, the cytomorphology of the tumour cells which are usually monomorphic throughout the lesion, and the presence of melanin pigment both in tumour cells and in macrophages. The lesion can be distinguished from malignant melanoma in most cases by the lack of intraepidermal spread of tumour cells, the symmetry of the lesion and the lack of intralesional transformation (Fig. 7.13). In addition, most pigmented spindle cell tumours are superficial, rarely extending deeply into the reticular dermis.

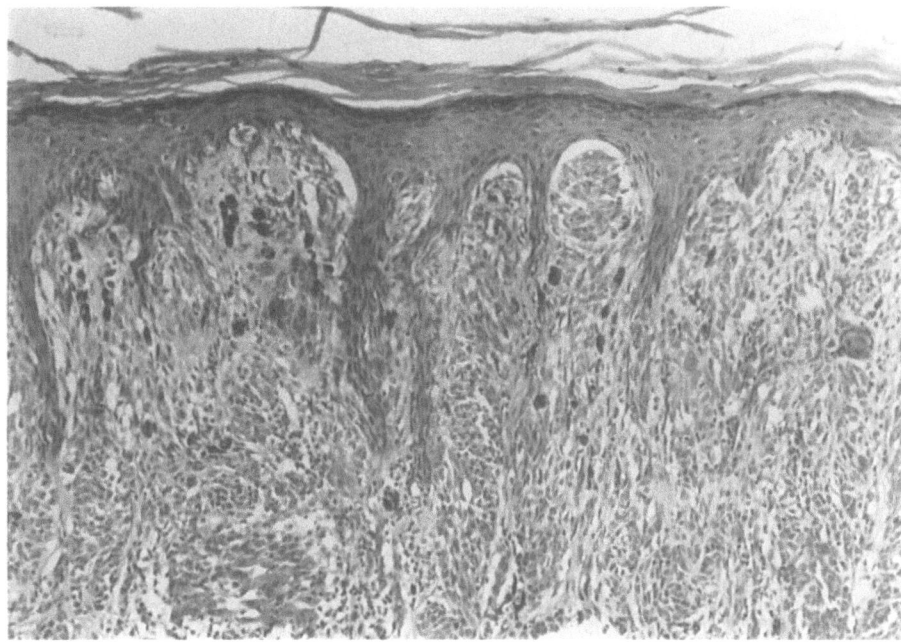

Fig. 7.11. Medium power view of the superficial portion of a pigmented spindle cell tumour. Note the almost continuous junctional component and numerous spindle cells and macrophages containing melanin.

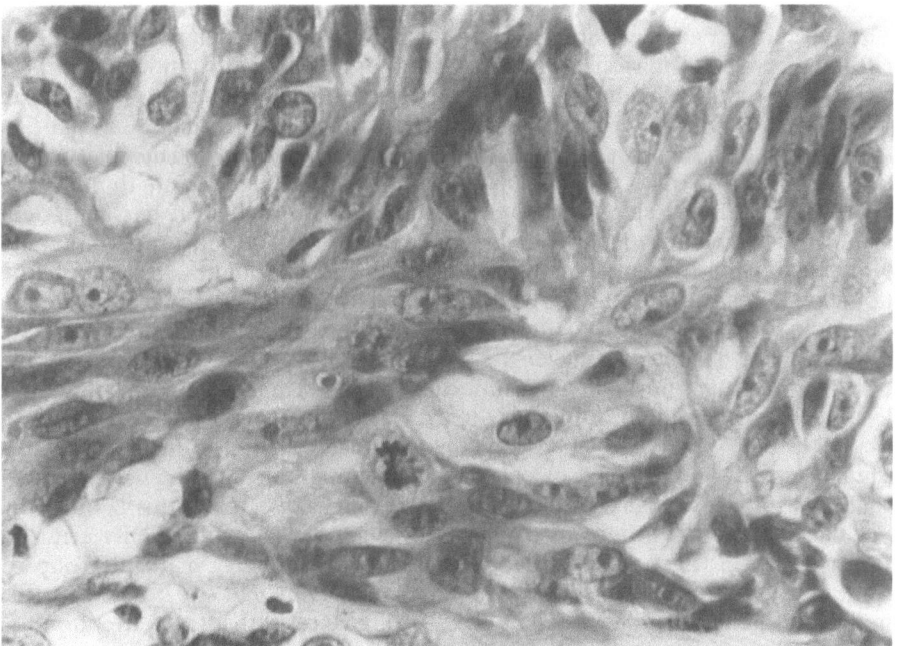

Fig. 7.12. Mitotic figures present in an area of a pigmented spindle cell tumour.

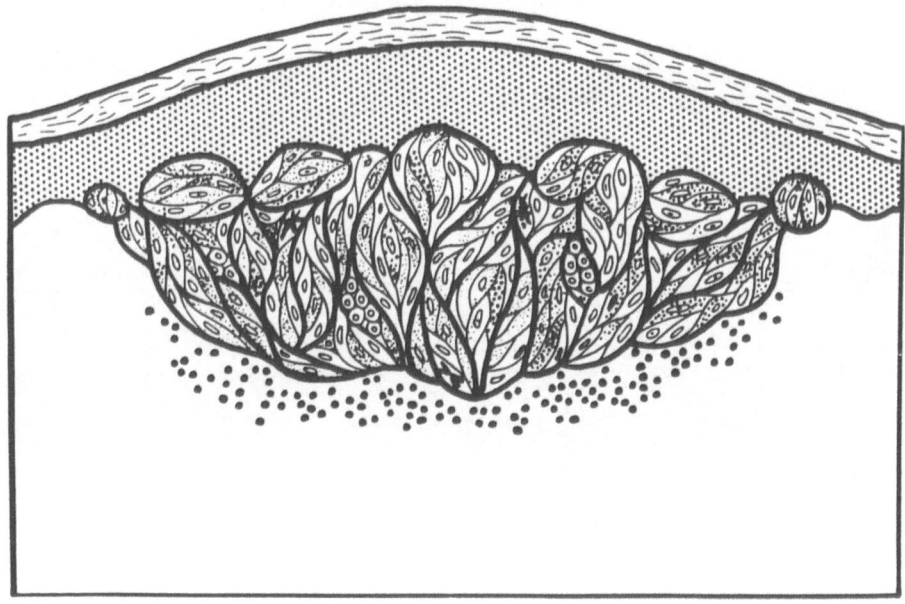

Fig. 7.13. Diagrammatic representation of the pathology of a typical pigmented spindle cell tumour. Reproduced from Smith (1987), with permission.

Halo Naevus (Sutton's Naevus) (Frank and Cohen 1964; Wayte and Helwig 1968)

The typical halo naevus is much easier for the clinician to diagnose than for the pathologist. The lesions, like many of the other melanocytic tumours discussed, are commoner in the young than the older age group and may be multiple. A pale halo develops around a pre-existing pigmented melanocytic naevus and in time the central pigmented area tends to disappear completely. The microscopic appearances of a halo naevus vary considerably depending on the stage of development of the lesion. Low power examination normally reveals a compound symmetrical melanocytic tumour associated with a very heavy predominantly lymphocytic infiltrate surrounding and extending throughout the lesion breaking up individual groups of tumour cells into small theques (Fig. 7.14). Some degree of cytological atypia in the tumour cells of a halo naevus may be seen and pyknotic and degenerate nuclei are not uncommon. Occasional mitoses may occur but these are normally not numerous. Of importance in differentiating this lesion from malignant melanoma is the overall low power symmetry of the lesion as well as the symmetry of the lymphocytic infiltrate. If it is difficult to visualize the naevus cells in the presence of a heavy infiltrate then labelling with a marker such as S100 can be very helpful (Figs. 7.15 and 7.16). When this is done one normally sees small groups of naevus cells symmetrically and evenly arranged throughout the lesion. If S100 labelling reveals asymmetry or focal groups of tumour cells with an expansile growth pattern it may be that one is dealing with a malignant melanoma, and Reed et al. (1990) have recently drawn attention to a halo naevus variant of minimum deviation malignant melanoma. It is sometimes useful to stain sections from a suspected halo naevus for melanin. In a typical

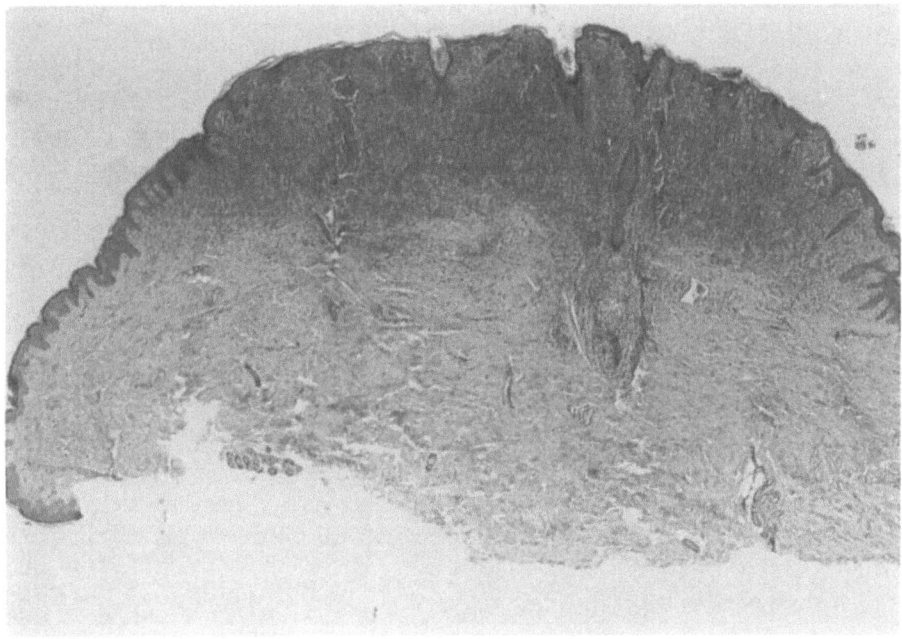

Fig. 7.14. Low power view of a halo naevus. Note the dense cellularity of the tumour and its bilateral symmetry.

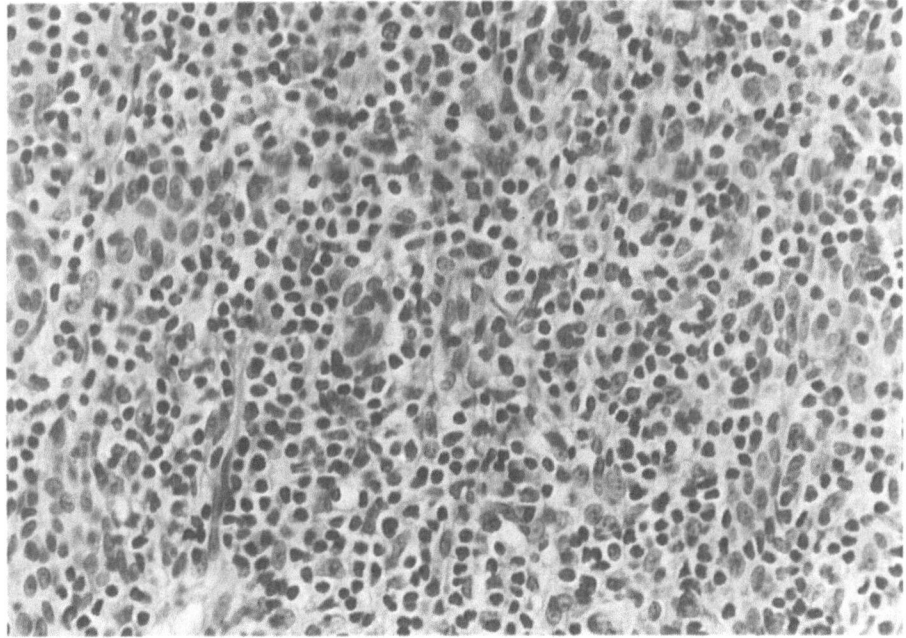

Fig. 7.15. Medium power view of a halo naevus. Individual tumour cells are broken up by a prominent lymphocytic infiltrate.

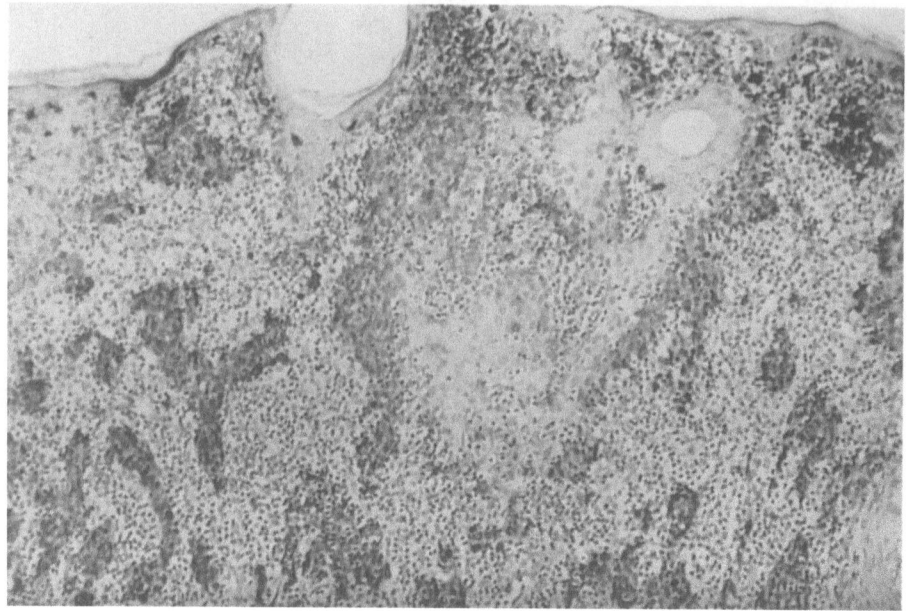

Fig. 7.16. Labelling with the S100 marker reveals small groups of naevus cells of equal size and distribution throughout the lesion.

lesion there is usually reduction in the normal melanin pigmentation of the lower layers of the epidermis on either side of the tumour. Although this is helpful it does not completely exclude melanoma as occasional malignant melanomas may also be surrounded by a depigmented halo. Clinicopathological correlation is most important in achieving a correct diagnosis with these lesions.

Recurrent Melanocytic Naevus Following Partial Surgical Removal ("Pseudomelanoma") (Kornberg and Ackerman 1975; Suster 1986)

Following the partial removal of a benign melanocytic naevus occasionally an irregularly pigmented area recurs in the biopsy site. This is particularly common following shave biopsies where deep naevus cells are left behind in the dermis. If these recurrent lesions are then excised and examined histologically certain atypical histopathological features may be noted, particularly in the superficial portions of the lesion. These may lead the pathologist to make an erroneous diagnosis of malignant melanoma in situ.

Low power examination usually reveals a proliferation of melanocytes at the epidermodermal junction with on occasion some degree of spread of tumour cells into the lower layers of the epidermis. the architectural pattern of junctional proliferation as well as the cytology of the proliferating cells may be atypical. In the underlying dermis there is usually some evidence of fibrosis indicating previous trauma or surgery. Deep to this area of fibrosis there may be residual mature intradermal naevus cells (Fig. 7.17a, b). Helpful points in differentiating

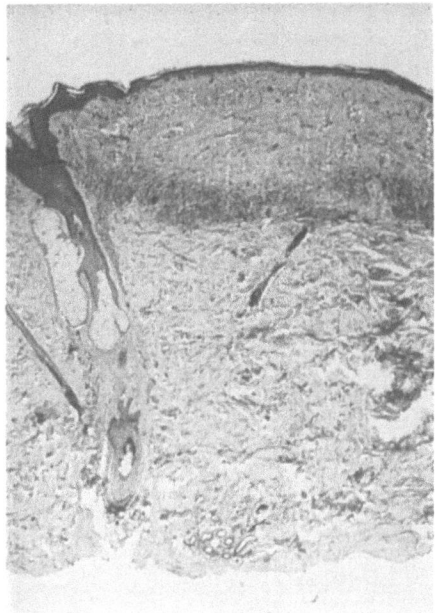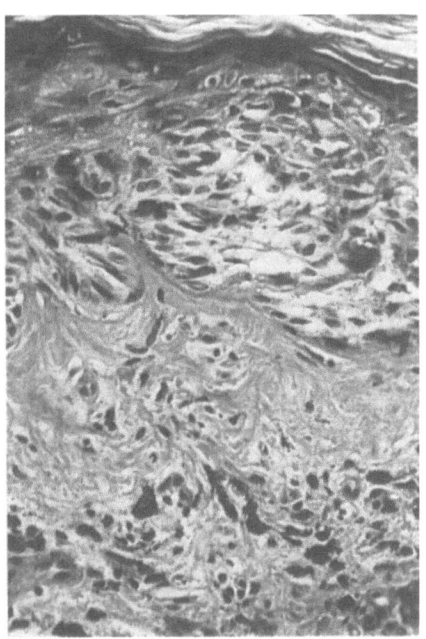

Fig. 7.17. a Low power view of recurrent naevus following shave biopsy. **b** Medium power view illustrating the atypical junctional component and dermal fibrosis.

this recurrent naevus from an in situ or early invasive malignant melanoma include:

1. Sharp lateral circumscription of the lesion
2. Atypical melanocytes confined to the junctional and superficial portion of the lesion
3. Atypical junctional melanocytes not extending laterally beyond the boundaries of the dermal fibrosis
4. (When present) naevus cells in the underlying dermis

It is obviously important for the clinician when re-excising a lesion which has recurred following partial surgical excision to pass on this information to the pathologist.

Atypical Naevi Occurring on the Genital Skin of Young Adults and on Acral Sites (Friedman and Ackerman 1981; Christensen et al. 1987)

In recent years it has been recognized that naevi occurring on certain sites, particularly pigmented naevi occurring on the vulval skin and occasionally on the skin of the shaft of the penis in young adults, may show unusual histological features. The histological features that may mimic melanoma are confined to the

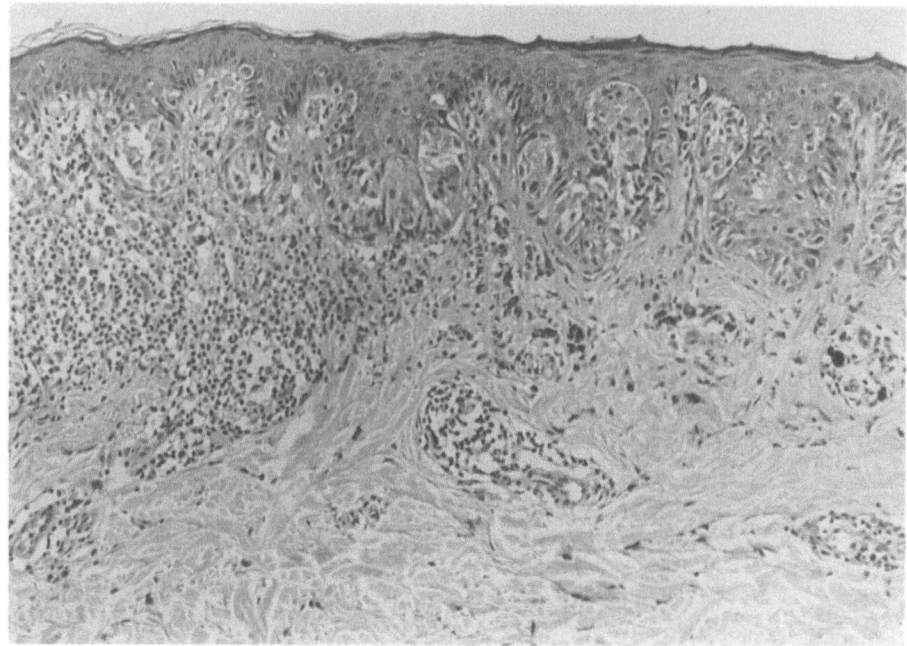

Fig. 7.18. A predominantly junctional naevus from the vulva of a 21-year-old female. Note the mild cytological and architectural atypia.

intraepidermal and junctional melanocytes (Fig. 7.18). An extensive junctional component is commonly seen. Individual tumour cells and groups of tumour cells vary in size and shape and the groups of tumour cells are not spaced equidistantly along the epidermodermal junction. Some confluence of tumour cell nests and extension of tumour cells down adnexal epithelium may be present. These histological features are not dissimilar to those sometimes observed in dysplastic naevi. Helpful points in differentiating naevi occurring on genital skin from malignant melanoma include sharp lateral demarcation, the presence of maturation with typical naevus cells in the underlying dermis, and the presence of cytological and architectural atypia confined to the superficial portion of the lesion.

Pigmented melanocytic naevi occurring on the skin of the palms and soles may also on occasion give rise to confusion. It should be remembered that even with naevi occurring in adults on these sites a prominent junctional component is frequently seen. In addition large dendritic melanocytes similar to those seen in acral lentiginous melanoma may be identified. However, as in the naevi discussed above, the dermal component of acral naevi shows little or no evidence of nuclear and cytological abnormality and mitotic figures are not normally seen. There is no convincing evidence that naevi of this type on the palms and soles are precursor lesions to melanoma but the myth that such lesions are in some way sinister is commonly encountered.

Deep Penetrating Naevus

In 1989 (Seab et al.) a series of 70 cases of heavily pigmented melanocytic naevi occurring particularly on the face, upper trunk and limbs was reported from the Armed Forces Institute of Pathology. The lesions occurred in children and young adults with an age range of 10–30 years. Despite an initial histological diagnosis of malignant melanoma in over a quarter of the cases no evidence of distant metastases or local recurrence was noted over a mean follow-up period of seven years. Microscopic examination of lesions of deep penetrating naevus revealed loosely arranged islands and fascicles of often heavily pigmented naevus cells extending deeply into the dermis and sometimes the subcutaneous tissues. In many lesions large numbers of melanin-containing macrophages were also seen. Many of the lesions had a wedge-shaped low power architecture and the junctional component was often not prominent and composed of small nests of cells. A lymphocytic host response was either absent or slight and tumour cells commonly extended around adnexal structures, blood vessels and nerves. In some cases pilomotor muscles were also infiltrated by tumour cells. High power examination revealed, in a number of cases, a moderate degree of cellular and nuclear pleomorphism. However, mitotic figures were not a feature of deep penetrating naevus. Although the lesion shows some features in common with some varieties of cellular blue naevus, the junctional component, which was commonly seen in deep penetrating naevus, as well as the absence of nests of non-pigmented or sparsely pigmented spindle cells aid in the differentiation of these two tumours. In very heavily pigmented examples of deep penetrating naevus distinction needs to be made from the unusual melanoma variant described by Wallace Clark as "animal"-type melanoma (oral presentation, American Society of Dermatopathology 1988; personal communication 1991). These tumours have been experimentally induced in guinea pigs and in humans, although the biological behaviour of "animal"-type melanoma is unpredictable, some examples have metastasized to regional lymph nodes. Whether deep penetrating naevus really is a specific entity or whether it is related on the one hand, to some forms of blue naevus or on the other hand to deep variants of pigmented spindle cell naevi, remains to be seen. It is also possible that a small number of these lesions may represent a form of minimum deviation melanoma and careful long-term clinical follow-up is recommended following the diagnosis of deep penetrating naevus.

Combined Melanocytic Naevi (Gartmann and Müller 1977; Rogers et al. 1985)

Occasionally melanocytic proliferations showing different histological features in different areas of the tumour may be encountered. The common combinations are between Spitz naevi, benign junctional and compound cellular naevi and blue naevi. The presence of some degree of cytological atypia and the low power architectural asymmetry may confuse the pathologist but the individual components of a combined naevus show the typical features that one normally associates with simple blue naevi, Spitz naevi or other benign melanocytic tumours.

Congenital Naevi (Mark et al. 1973; Silvers and Helwig 1981)

The unusual histological features that may occur in congenital naevi include variation in pattern and cytology in the deeper parts of the lesion where on occasion expansile nests of tumour cells are found which show different characteristics from naevus cells elsewhere in the tumour. This feature can simulate so-called intralesional transformation which is normally only seen in the vertical growth phase of invasive malignant melanoma. In congenital melanocytic naevi biopsied very shortly after birth, the junctional and superficial portion of the naevus frequently shows atypical features. Nests of melanocytes of variable size and shape are seen at the epidermodermal junction. Furthermore, individual melanocytes may be seen at levels higher in the epidermis, even on occasions reaching the cornified layer. The presence of naevus cells in the deeper tissues with a tumour cell cytomorphology and an architectural arrangement character- istic for congenital naevus, is crucial to the correct diagnosis.

Pagetoid and Balloon Naevus Cells in Naevi (Wilson Jones and Sanderson 1963; Schrader and Helwig 1967)

The term pagetoid naevus cells has been used to describe large cells with abundant pale-staining cytoplasm often containing finely dispersed melanin pigment. Balloon cells tend to be even larger with clear cytoplasm. Focal balloon cell or pagetoid cell change within what appear to be benign cellular naevi, is not an uncommon histological variation (Fig. 7.19). It is unusual, however, to encounter a melanocytic naevus composed almost entirely of such cells. The size

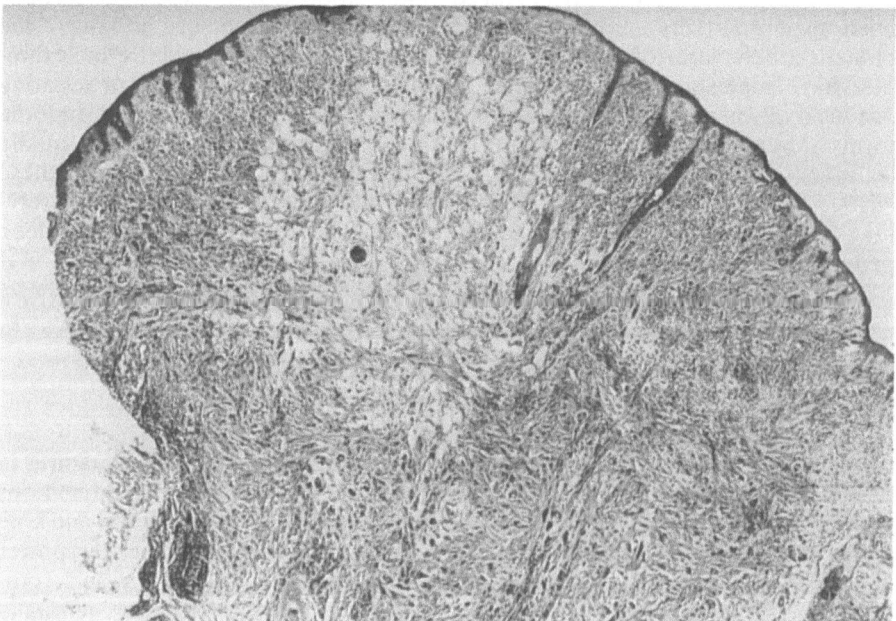

Fig. 7.19.   Focal balloon cell change in a benign compound cellular naevus.

of the cells and the resemblance of some pagetoid cells to those seen in invasive malignant melanoma can give cause for concern. However, mitotic figures and nuclear atypia is not seen in the benign lesions and normally in superficial spreading (pagetoid) melanoma, pagetoid melanoma cells are almost always seen at the epidermodermal junction and within the epidermis in addition to in the dermal component.

"Ancient" Naevi

It has recently been reported that in some naevi removed from middle-aged and elderly patients, some degree of cell atypia may lead to an erroneous diagnosis of malignant melanoma. In these lesions haemorrhage is frequently prominent and the cytological and nuclear abnormalities that may be seen in focal areas are presumably associated with a form of involutional change. The presence of mitotic figures in such lesions, particularly if they are numerous or atypical, is likely to indicate that the lesion is a melanoma and not an example of so-called ancient naevus.

Dysplastic Naevi

The concepts of dysplastic naevi and dysplastic naevus syndrome continue to excite controversy among dermatopathologists (Elder et al. 1982; Roth et al. 1991). One of the problems is that the clinical criteria for such lesions, such as size >6 mm, a prominent macular component, irregular and indistinct margins, and variability of pigmentation within the lesion often with a prominent reddish or tan colour, do not correlate well with the histological criteria used for a diagnosis of dysplastic naevi. Furthermore, various pathologists use different criteria for the histological diagnosis of dysplastic naevi. In the writings of Wallace Clark and David Elder the histopathological criteria for the diagnosis of dysplastic naevi have been clearly set out. Although there have been minor changes and refinements made by these authors to the criteria over the years with increased experience, the basic diagnostic features for such lesions remain the same. These include some evidence of architectural atypia of the proliferating melanocytic component, particularly at the epidermodermal junction, and at least some degree of cytological atypia (Fig. 7.20). In addition, there is evidence of a cellular and mesenchymal host response with a chronic inflammatory cell infiltrate in the subjacent dermis as well as some evidence of fibrosis. It has been suggested that it might be better to abandon the term dysplastic naevi and substitute a descriptive report based on the above features (Seywright et al. 1985). This suggestion has the merit of facilitating communication between pathologists and avoids the ambiguity with which the term dysplastic naevus is nowadays regarded. The only malignant melanoma which is likely to be confused with a dysplastic naevus is a melanoma that is either in situ or only invading the papillary dermis. If one agrees with Clark's hypothesis of tumour development (Herlyn et al. 1987), lesions not in the vertical growth phase are incapable of metastasis and

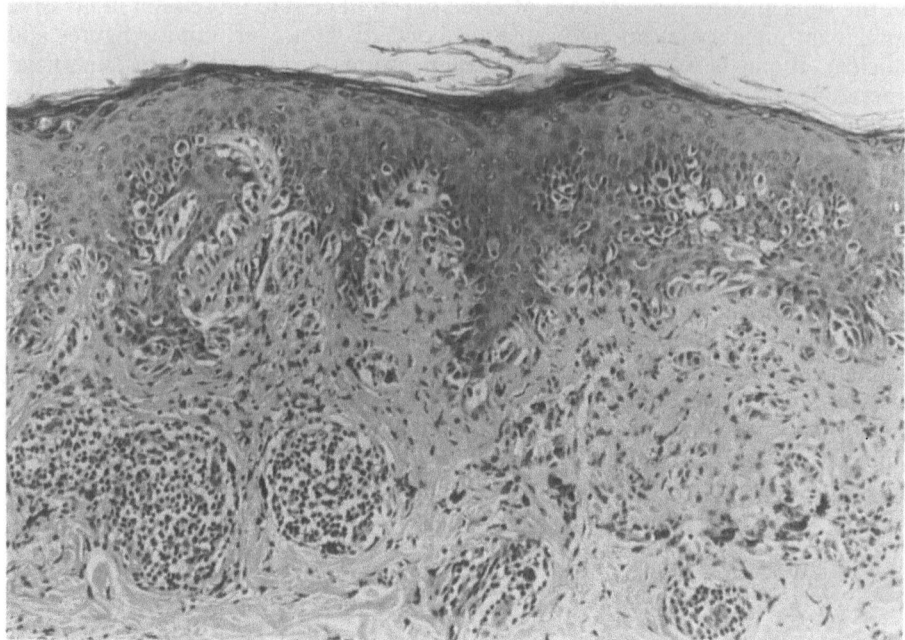

Fig. 7.20. Example of a dysplastic naevus. Note the cytological and architectural atypia of melanocytic proliferation with elongation of rete ridges, dermal fibrosis and a patchy chronic inflammatory cell host response.

therefore in one sense are not even truly malignant. Superficial lesions with architectural and cytological atypia, once they have been completely excised are cured, and because of this they pose less of a problem for both the clinician and the diagnostic histopathologist than large atypical melanocytic lesions with a deep dermal component.

Conclusions

It is clear from the comments above that the most important prerequisites for an accurate diagnosis of a benign melanocytic lesion and its differentiation from malignant melanoma are close co-operation between the clinician and the pathologist and the awareness on the part of the pathologist of the wide spectrum of different benign melanocytic tumours that may on occasions simulate a malignant melanoma. In achieving an accurate diagnosis we not only directly benefit our patients but we improve the accuracy of accumulated data on the biology of malignant melanoma. At the same time it is most important to realize that some lesions have histopathological features that are impossible to force into a specific diagnostic category. In these cases descriptive histological reporting and long-term careful clinical follow-up may lead to the description of new clinicopathological entities and will increase our understanding of the rich variety of melanocytic tumours and their behaviour.

References

Amazon K, Robinson MJ, Rywlin AM (1980) Ferrugination caused by Monsel's solution. Am J Dermatopathol 2:197–205

Barnhill RL, Mihm MC (1989) Pigmented spindle cell naevus and its variants: distinction from melanoma. Br J Dermatol 121:717–726

Barr RJ, Morales RV, Graham JH (1980) Desmoplastic nevus. A distinct variant of mixed spindle cell and epithelioid cell nevus. Cancer 46:557–564

Bourlond A (1971) Multiple juvenile melanoma. Hautarzt 4:144–149

Brownstein WE (1972) Multiple agminated juvenile melanoma. Arch Dermatol 106:89–91

Christensen WN, Friedman KJ, Woodruff JD, Hood AF (1987) Histologic characteristics of vulvlar nevocellular nevi. J Cutan Pathol 14:87–91

Coskey RJ, Mehregan A (1973) Spindle cell nevi in adults and children. Arch Dermatol 108:535–536

Echevarria R, Ackerman LV (1967) Spindle and epithelioid cell nevi in the adult. Cancer 20:175–189

Elder DE, Green MH, Guerry D, Kraemer KH, Clark WH (1982) The dysplastic nevus syndrome. Am J Dermatopathol 4:455–460

Frank SB, Cohen HJ (1964) The halo naevus. Arch Dermatol 89:367–373

Friedman RJ, Ackerman AB (1981) Difficulties in the histologic diagnosis of melanocytic nevi on the vulvae of premenopausal women. In: Ackerman AB (ed.) Pathology of malignant melanoma. Masson, New York, pp 119–127

Gartmann H (1980) Der pigmentierte Spindelzellentumor (PSCT). Z Hautkr 56:862–876

Gartmann H, Ganser M (1984) Der Spitz-Naevus. Spindelzellen- und/oder Epitheloidzellennaevus – Eine histologische Analyse von 652 Tumoren. Z Hautkr 60:29–42

Gartmann H, Müller HD (1977) Über das gemeinsame Vorkommen von blauem Naevus und Naevuszellnaevus. Z Hautkr 52:389–398

Gould DJ, Bleehen SS (1980) Multiple agminate juvenile melanoma. Clin Exp Dermatol 5:63–65

Herlyn M, Clark WH, Rodeck U, Manciani ML, Jambrosic J, Koprowski H (1987) Biology of tumour progression in human melanocytes. Lab Invest 56:461–474

Kamino H, Misheloff E, Ackerman AB, Flotte TJ, Greco MA (1979) Eosinophilic globules in Spitz's nevi. Am J Dermatopathol 1:319–324

Kornberg R, Ackerman AB (1975) Pseudomelanoma. Recurrent melanocytic nevus following partial surgical removal. Arch Dermatol 111: 1588–1590

Lancer HA, Muhlbauer JE, Sober AJ (1983) Multiple agminated spindle cell nevi: unique clinical presentation and review. J Am Acad Dermatol 8:707–711

Liftin AJ, Schwarz R, Jagirdar J (1985) Fibronectin-containing hyaline globules in malignant melanoma. Am J Dermatopathol 7:17–21

Mark GJ, Mihm MC Jr, Liteplo MG, Reed RJ, Clark WH (1973) Congenital melanocytic nevi of the small and garment type. Hum Pathol 4:395–418

Michie SA, Abel EA, Hoppe RT, Warnke RA, Wood GS (1990) Discordant expression of antigens between intraepidermal and intradermal T cells in mycosis fungoides. Am J Pathol 137:1447–1451

Mishima Y, Pinkus H (1960) Benign mixed tumor of melanocytes and Malpighian cells. Arch Dermatol 81:539–550

Olmstead PM, Lund HZ, Leonard DD (1980) Monsel's solution: a histologic nuisance. J Am Acad Dermatol 3:492–498

Paniago-Pereira C, Maize JC, Ackerman AB (1978) Nevus of large spindle and/or epithelioid cells (Spitz's nevus). Arch Dermatol 114:1811–1823

Reed RJ, Ichinose H, Clark WH et al. (1975) Common and uncommon melanocytic nevi and borderline melanomas. Semin Oncol 2:119–147

Reed RJ, Webb SV, Clark WH Jr (1990) Minimal deviation melanoma: halo naevus variant. Am J Surg Pathol 14:53–68

Rogers G, Advani H, Ackerman AB (1985) A combined variant of Spitz's nevi: how to differentiate them from malignant melanomas. Am J Dermatopathol 7:61–78

Roth ME, Grant-Kels JM, Ackerman AB, Elder DE, Friedman RJ, Heilman ER, Maize JC, Sagebiel
RW (1991) The histopathology of dysplastic nevi. Am J Dermatopathol 13:38–51
Sagebiel RW, Chinn EK, Egbert BM (1984) Pigmented spindle cell nevus: clinical and histologic
review of 90 cases. Am J Surg Pathol 8:645–653
Schrader WA, Helwig EB (1967) Balloon cell nevi. Cancer 20:1502–1514
Seab JA, Graham JH, Helwig EB (1989) Deep penetrating nevus. Am J Surg Pathol 13:39–44
Seywright MM, Doherty VR, MacKie RM (1985) Proposed alternative terminology and subclassifi-
cation of so called "dysplastic naevi". J Clin Pathol 39:189–194
Silvers DN, Helwig EB (1981) Melanocytic nevi in neonates. J Am Acad Dermatol 4:166–175
Smith NP (1987) The pigmented spindle cell tumour of Reed: an underdiagnosed lesion. Semin Diagn
Pathol 4:75–87
Spitz S (1948) Melanomas of childhood. Am J Pathol 24:591–609
Suster S (1986) Pseudomelanoma. A pathologist's perspective. Int J Dermatol 25:506–507
Wayte DM, Helwig EB (1968) Halo nevi. Cancer 22:69–90
Wilson Jones E. Sanderson KV (1963) Cellular naevi with peculiar foam cells. Br J Dermatol 75:47–54
Wilson Jones E, Cerio R, Smith NP (1989) Epithelioid cell histiocytoma: a new entity. Br J Dermatol
120:185–195
Wood C, Severin GL (1980) Unusual histiocytic reaction to Monsel's solution. Am J Dermatopathol
2:261·264

8   Prognostic Factors in Melanoma

Michele M. Delaunay

Substantial advances have been made in the definition of prognostic factors in melanoma, with such precision that mathematical models have been established to predict individual survival (Soong 1985). The definition of prognostically important factors has had a practical impact. On the individual level, this makes it possible accurately to define therapeutic options and follow up schedules. On a more general level it allows for the definition of coherent groups in order to stratify therapeutic trials and analyse their results. Moreover, prognostic factors may provide information, or at least raise more questions, about the biology and natural history of melanoma.

An initial difficulty in the analysis of prognostic factors is the heterogeneity of the patient groups and of the definitions used in the numerous published studies on the subject. Reference criteria are not always the same. Definitions of 5- or 10-year survival rates, disease-free survival, remission over five years, and so on, vary from study to study. Usually patients are included at the stage of first admission to a medical centre, but the data used may also come from a national or regional cancer register. Two levels of analysis are possible; univariate, where each factor is separately analysed; multivariate, where factors are analysed in sequence to determine the predictive value of each variable taken alone and together with the others (Table 8.2). Finally, there are some factors which can not or can only partially be analysed, but must be taken into consideration.

As in all cancers, the first point to consider is the stage of the disease, which is established after appropriate staging investigations. In the case of melanoma these are restricted to a complete physical examination and a baseline chest X-ray. Chances of survival and prognostic factors are completely different in each stage. In the discussion of stages that follows, the M.D. Anderson classification will be used.

Localized Melanoma (Stage I) (Tables 8.1 and 8.2)

Tumour thickness is so important in this stage that most other factors seem to correlate with it, but this correlation is not complete (i.e. not all factors are

Table 8.1. Prognostic factors in Stage I

Parameters	Analysis		Main references
	Single fact	Multifact	
Clinical			
Stage	++++	++++	
Sex	+++	++	Blois et al. (1983a); Cascinelli et al. (1980); Drzewiecki and Andersen (1982); Johnson et al. (1985); Levy et al. (1991); O'Doherty et al. (1986); Schmoeckel et al. (1983); Shaw et al. (1980a); Weidner (1981)
Age	++	−	Balch et al. (1979, 1985); Levy et al. (1991)
Sex/age	++	+	Levy et al. (1991); Maize (1983)
Hormonal status	+		Meyskens et al. (1988); Shaw et al. (1980a, b)
Initial site	+++	+	Balch et al. (1985); Blois et al. (1983b); Clark et al. (1989); Day et al. (1982a, b); Drzewiecki and Andersen (1982); Weidner (1981)
Race	++	− (?)	Sober (1989)
Pathological and other			
Tumour thickness	+++	+++	Berdeaux et al. (1989); Blois et al. (1983a, b); Braun-Falco et al. (1986); Cascinelli et al. (1980); Drzewiecki et al. (1990); Elias et al. (1977); Johnson et al. (1985); Karakousis et al. (1989); Karjalainen and Hakulinen (1988); Kelly et al. (1985b); Kopf et al. (1987a); Kuehnl-Petzoldt et al. (1983); Lee (1980); Lemish et al. (1981); McGovern et al. (1983); Palangie et al. (1981); Sober (1989); Sober et al. (1983a, b); Stolz et al. (1989); van der Esch et al. (1981)
Level	++	+	
Ulceration	++	+	Balch et al. (1980); Drzewiecki and Andersen (1982); Kuehnl-Petzoldt et al. (1983)
Histogenetic type	++	+/−	Clark et al. (1989); Day et al. (1982c); van der Esch et al. (1981)
Mitotic and prognostic index	++ ++	+ ++	Kopf et al. (1987a); Schmoeckel et al. (1983); Stolz et al. (1989); van der Esch et al. (1981)
Regression	+/−		Clark et al. (1989); MacKie et al. (1991); Shaw et al. (1989); Slingluff et al. (1988); Trau et al. (1983)
Pigmentation	+	?	Balch et al. (1985)
Cellular type	+		Drzewiecki and Andersen (1982); van der Esch et al. (1981)
Lymphocytic infiltration, TIL	+		Clark et al. (1989); Day et al. (1982c)
Inflammatory response			van der Esch et al. (1981)
Microsatellitosis			Day et al. (1982b)
Angioinvasion			van der Esch et al. (1981)

Table 8.1. *continued*

Parameters	Analysis		Main references
	Single fact	Multifact	
Oncogenes Chromosomal abnormalities	+		Funasaka et al. (1988); Pierard (1988)
Varia			
Immunological factors	?		Clark et al. (1989)
Psychological factors Social conditions	+	N/A	Cassileth et al. (1982); Rogentine et al. (1979); Shaw and Milton (1981); Temoshok et al. (1985)
Therapeutics			
Initial assessment, follow up counselling	+	N/A	Johnson et al. (1985)
Excision margins	++		
Elective node dissection	+	+/−	Balch et al. (1985); Day et al. (1982c)
Adjuvant therapy	−		

++++ All other factors analysed for Stage 1.
+++ Significant in all studies
++   Significant in most studies
+   Significant in some studies
−   Non significant
N/A Not analysable

concerned) or total (i.e. some factors are independent in definite subgroups of thickness, or after exclusion of thin tumours) (Balch et al. 1979, 1985; Griffel 1981, Day et al. 1982, a, b, c; Day et al. 1983; Griffiths and Briggs 1984) (Table 8.3).

Histopathological Factors

Breslow Thickness

Thickness as defined by Breslow is decisive; this underlines the importance of the technical conditions of its measurement. Thickness determines all aspects of tumour evolution: (a) risk of metastases and risk of death; (b) time to recurrence and survival; (c) type of first recurrence.

Risk of death is measured by 5- or 10-year survival rate (these differ by 5–10 points). The relationship between thickness and survival is progressive but not continuous especially at the extremes: under 0.76 mm thick, more than 95% of the tumours are curable; over 5 to 6 mm thick, most tumours are fatal. Karakousis et al. (1989) has measured this progression for 371 Stage I melanomas. Over 1 mm, for each 1 mm increment in thickness, the survival rate declines in women by about 3% up to 6 mm and by about 8% in the range of 7–15 mm of thickness. For men the survival rate declines by about 9% per mm up to 10 mm.

Table 8.2. Independent prognostic factors: main multifactorial analysis (1979–1990)

	Cascinelli et al. (1980)	Johnson et al. (1985)	Worth et al. (1989)	Blois et al. (1983a)	Tonak (1985)	Meyskens et al. (1988)	Berdeaux et al. (1989)	Balch et al. (1985)	Drzewiecki et al. (1990)	Cox (1985)	Clark et al. (1989)	Kopf (1987b)
Number of patients	747	262	798	1123	455	377	259	3505	714	1071	386	879
	Thickness		Thickness (log)	Thickness	Thickness	Thickness	Thickness	Thickness	Histogenetic	Mitotic type	Prognostic index	Prognostic index
	Sex		Sex (<4mm)	Sex		Sex/age	Pathological stage	ELND	Ulceration	Thickness	TIL	Thickness
				Site		Ulceration	Sex/age	Site	Epithelioid cells	Ulceration	Thickness	Ulceration
						ELND		Ulceration	Sex	Site	Site	Site
								Pathological stage[a]	Site		Regression	Age
								Level[b]	Inflammatory infiltration		Sex	
								Sex[b]				
								Regression[b]				

[a] Pathological node involvement after elective node dissection (ELND).
[b] Independent factor only in subgroups.

Table 8.3. Prognostic factors in three groups of thickness subsets

Thickness	0.76 → 1.69 mm	1.51 → 3.99 mm	> 3.65 mm
Number of patients	203	177	79
Independent factors (multivariate analysis of 14 parameters)	Site BANS Non-BANS[a]	Mitoses > 6/mm^2 Site Ulceration > 3 mm Microsatellitosis	Lymphocytic response Histogenetic type (non-SSM) Site (trunk) Pathological Stage III[b]

From Day et al. (1982a).
[a] Back, arm, neck, scalp.
[b] Pathological node involvement after elective node dissection.

It is interesting that this progressive correlation is not continuous at the extremes and especially for thin tumours. This raises the question of the significance of vertical and radial growth phases, where the radial growth phase is said to have a very limited metastatic potential. Moreover, it questions the definition of prognostic groups defined by strict division into subsets by thickness alone, which are necessary for example to compare two therapeutic decisions (in the group of thickness 1.5–4 mm, recurrence and survival rates are very different at the extremes).

Thickness is a predictive factor of remission and duration of survival. Thick tumours recur sooner (mean disease-free interval is 3.5 years between 1 and 2 mm, 2 years between 3 and 4 mm, 1.4 years between 4 and 5 mm) (Kelly et al. 1985a) (Table 8.4). As a major indicator of both disease-free interval and risk of

Table 8.4. Annual risk of recurrence according to thickness

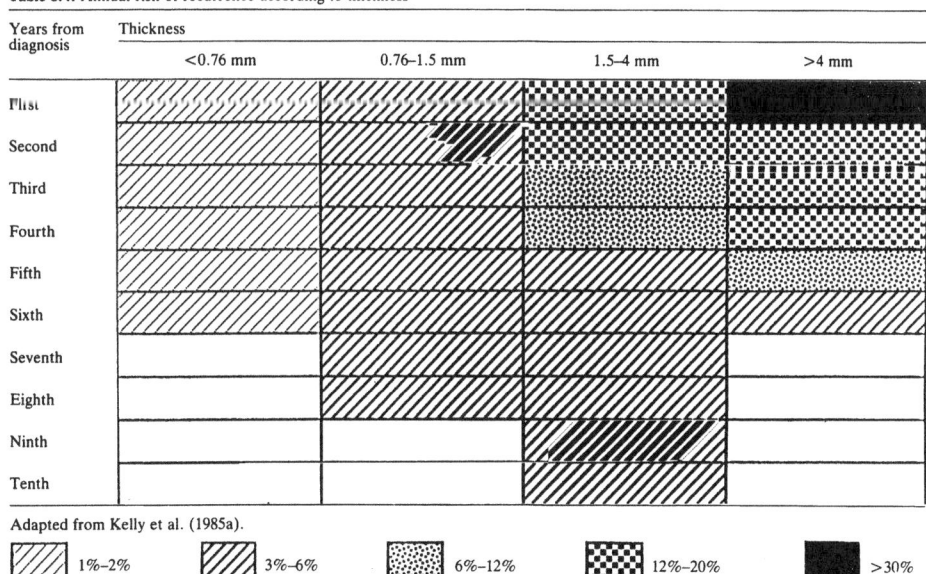

Adapted from Kelly et al. (1985a).

Table 8.4. Annual risk of recurrence according to thickness

recurrence, thickness can be used in designing follow-up schedules. As thickness increases, survival time decreases. the "hazard rate of death" (probability of dying per unit of time) peaks at 72 months for melanomas <0.75 mm thick; 60 months between 1.51 and 3 mm; 48 months between 1.51 and 3 mm; and 40 months >3 mm (Rogers et al. 1986).

The site of recurrence is also influenced by tumour thickness. Risk of local recurrence correlates directly with thickness: less than 0.5% under 0.76 mm; more than 10% above 4 mm (Balch et al. 1979). Regional metastases are proportionately more frequent for thick tumours and this is apparent in the series of Balch and Milton as a difference in mean thickness of primary tumours in Stage III (regional) (3.5 mm) and in Stage IV (distant metastases) (2.7 mm) (Balch et al. 1985).

Level of Invasion

Level of invasion has no additional prognostic value after thickness has been considered, except in the case of thin melanomas (Kelly et al. 1985b) and in one study of tumours over 4 mm (Soong 1985). An independent pejorative predictive value of level V has not been demonstrated.

Ulceration

The presence of ulceration has been found to be a significant negative factor in several studies (Balch et al. 1980; Meyskens et al. 1988) and is more pejorative the greater its extent (>6 mm diameter) (Balch et al. 1980).

Histogenetic Type and Growth Pattern

The significance of histogenetic type, which is supposed to indicate a radial or vertical growth pattern, is still controversial. When patients with superficial spreading melanoma and nodular melanoma are matched for thickness, no difference in survival is found.

Depending on the studies, patients with lentigo maligna melanoma have (Balch et al. 1985) or do not have (McGovern et al. 1983) a better prognosis. No clear difference in survival has been found for acral lentiginous melanoma (Sondergaard and Olsen 1980; Krementz et al. 1982). The controversy persists between those who make no difference between melanoma types whatever the site (Ackerman 1982) and those who establish a prognostic limit between radial and vertical growth (Clark). In a recent study of 386 cases, all patients with tumours considered in radial growth phase survived without evidence of disease for a minimum of 8 years (Clark et al. 1989).

Mitotic Index and Prognostic Index

Prognostic index as reported by Schmoeckel et al. (1983) (thickness × mitotic index, i.e. number of mitoses/mm^2) enhances the predictive value of thickness especially between 1.5 and 4 mm (Kopf et al. 1987a).

Other Histoprognostic Factors

Some other histoprognostic factors are discussed in the literature. Regression (the definition of which is somewhat subjective) may lead to an underestimation of Breslow thickness and can be associated with an unfavourable prognosis of thin tumours (Ronan et al. 1987; Slingluff et al. 1988; Shaw et al. 1989). This pejorative significance is not accepted by all authors (Balch et al. 1979, 1985; McGovern et al. 1983).

Lymphocytic infiltration is associated with better survival and may or may not correlate with thickness (Balch et al. 1985; Clark et al. 1989). Clark et al. had defined a prognostic model including the presence of tumour infiltrating lymphocytes and five other significant factors (mitotic rate, thickness, site, sex, histological regression) (Table 8.2). They consider that this system constitutes the most accurate approach in survival prediction (Clark et al. 1989).

Other parameters are occasionally analysed and are of secondary practical importance: pigmentation, cellular type, inflammatory response, angioinvasion, and the clinical presence of multiple primary tumours (van der Esch et al. 1981; Watzig and Knopf 1981; Day et al. 1982b; Drzewiecki and Andersen 1982; Balch et al. 1985; Clark et al. 1989; Gupta et al. 1991).

Non-histopathological Factors

Sex

Melanoma is the tumour in which gender most influences survival. In women, survival rates are higher by 8%–10% in Stage I and by 10%–15% in all other Stages. This difference is constant in all countries whatever the period of study (survival rates are 23.4% and 34.5% in 1901 cases reported between 1949 and 1959 and respectively 56.5% and 70% in 5738 cases reported between 1978 and 1983). Stability in prognostic difference contrasts with a general tendency to levelling out of incidence in men and women. The sex difference in survival is partly attributable to site and thickness (Shaw et al. 1980b) but nevertheless persists for tumours of identical location (Shaw et al. 1980a) and of equal thickness (Cascinelli et al. 1980; Drzewiecki and Andersen 1982; Blois et al. 1983a).

Several studies suggest a deterioration in prognosis in postmenopausal women and a consequently similar survival rate in men and women aged over 50 years (Shaw et al. 1980b, Meyskens et al. 1988). This suggests that hormonal status is of some relevance. The same is also conceivable for pregnancy: statistically it is not noticeable (MacKie et al. 1991) but one cannot exclude the possibility that pregnancy may have a pejorative influence on exceptional cases of melanoma, despite the absence of any conclusive study of steroid receptors for a possible variable hormonal dependence of the tumours.

In spite of the rarity of melanoma in childhood and the independent predictive value of gender the significance of sex steroids remains unclear and no decisive therapeutic role for them has yet been determined.

Anatomical Location of Primary Lesion

The prognostic importance of the initial site of the melanoma is of particular interest because the prognosis differs according to anatomical location and within different groups of thickness subsets.

When considering the major anatomical locations (head and neck, trunk, extremities), site may (Balch et al. 1979; Blois et al. 1983a; Soong 1985; Kopf et al. 1987b; Clark et al. 1989) or may not be (Cascinelli et al. 1980; van der Esch et al. 1981; Drzewiecki and Andersen 1982; Berdeaux et al. 1989; Worth et al. 1989) of independent prognostic significance. In the study by Balch and Milton (1985), this significance becomes apparent only after exclusion of tumours thinner than 0.76 mm: axial melanomas are more pejorative than melanomas on the limbs. Head and neck lesions have a rather similar prognosis to truncal lesions, being either slightly less favourable (Blois et al. 1983a) or slightly more favourable (Balch et al. 1985).

Analysis of anatomical subsites reveals further differences in prognosis. Generally speaking, prognosis is worse when the melanoma is situated closer to a greater number or groups of regional lymph nodes, with the notable exception of the hands and feet, and in only one study in the thigh compared to the leg (Rogers et al. 1986). Day et al. (1982a) attributed a pejorative significance to BANS lesions (lesions located in upper Back, posterior Arm, posterior Neck and posterior Scalp) in the group of thickness 0.76–1.69 mm (Table 8.3). This notion was later contested.

Patients with melanoma located on the hands and feet have a significantly worse prognosis than those with lesions on the arm or leg (Day et al. 1982b, c, Rogers et al. 1983; Balch et al. 1985). Including the hands and feet in the notion of extremities in most series is confusing and attenuates the prognostic difference from axial melanomas.

Specific subsites have often been found to have a pejorative significance. These include the scalp and ear in the head and neck region, strictly midline locations and, of these, mucosal locations. In vulvar melanoma for example, prognosis is worse in the median mucosal part and survival rates may vary by 100% according to the location on the labia majora or on the mucosa (Podratz et al. 1983) with maximal severity when the clitoris, vagina or urethra are involved. Overall, all mucous membrane melanomas are severe but their rarity precludes multifactorial analysis and the relative influence of histoprognostic factors, location and mucosal type cannot be assessed.

Age

Advanced age correlates with shortened survival, apparently because older patients present with thicker lesions, but in most studies age has no independent prognostic value.

Race

It is almost impossible to assess the eventual prognostic difference according to race; in black and in Chinese and Japanese patients, melanoma is an aggressive malignancy with a high mortality rate since tumours occur predominantly on the extremities or mucosal sites and are usually thicker and more often ulcerated because they are more often diagnosed at an advanced stage.

The prognosis of melanomas located on the hands and feet in Japanese patients and white Americans seems to be similar but the number of cases reported is too small to allow any definitive conclusion (Sober 1989).

Other Factors

Therapeutic parameters are, of course, fundamental but cannot often be directly analysed. Observation of adequate margins of excision influences risk of local recurrence and metastatic risk, although the latter has been less precisely studied (Gutman et al. 1989). Elective node dissection has, in two North American studies (Balch et al. 1985; Meyskens et al. 1988), been found to be one of four independent prognostic variables, although other studies such as the WHO randomized prospective trial demonstrated no survival difference between prophylactic and therapeutic node dissection (at least in precisely defined conditions of follow-up). No adjuvant therapy has yet been demonstrated to be of any benefit.

Initial assessment, counselling and follow-up must be taken into consideration although they cannot be directly analysed. Five-year survival rate is 75% versus 43% in the series from Roswell Park Memorial Hospital depending on whether the initial treatment was in the medical centre or not, but the two groups were not completely comparable (Johnson et al. 1985). Many other parameters are not directly quantifiable, but should not be neglected all the same; such is the case with psychological factors (Rogentine et al. 1979; Temoshok et al. 1985), diet, smoking (Lemish et al. 1981; Shaw and Milton 1981) and social status.

Regional Nodal Melanoma (Stage IIIa) (Table 8.5)

Most disseminated melanomas go through a regional nodal stage at which, in most cases the disease may be curable. This fundamental notion in itself justifies follow-up.

The risk of recurrence of regional nodal melanoma is twice that of Stage I melanoma. It is also earlier and median remission time is less than one year (10.8 months in 200 patients from Balch; 10 months in 54 patients from Berdeaux) (Balch et al. 1985; Berdeaux et al. 1989). Overall 5-year survival is 20%–50% (Balch et al. 1985; Morton et al. 1985; Berdeaux et al. 1989) but the chances of survival are very different according to the degree of nodal involvement and the thickness of the initial tumour (Table 8.5).

Table 8.5 Prognostic factors in Stage IIIa (regional nodal)

Parameters	Significance	Main references
Tumour thickness	++	Balch et al.
Sex	+	(1979); Day et al.
Remission duration (I–III)	+	(1983); Morton
Number of metastatic nodes	+++	et al. (1985);
Capsular effraction	++	Roses et al.
Association of cutaneous regional metastases (Stage IIIb)	+	(1991)
Completeness of node dissection	+++	

Number of Metastatic Nodes

The number of metastatic nodes is very important (Cascinelli et al. 1980; Day et al. 1981; Balch et al. 1985; Morton et al. 1985; Berdeaux et al. 1989). Ten-year survival rate in 551 cases of regional nodal melanomas demonstrates that only patients with one positive node have a reasonable prospect of cure. Three years after diagnosis of nodal metastases, differences in survival are already statistically significant between groups with only one node, between two and four nodes and more than five nodes involved (Balch et al. 1985). The results of Morton et al.'s (1985) analysis are remarkably similar (Table 8.6). The extent of nodal metastases and capsular invasion have a significant impact on survival.

Table 8.6. Survival rates in Stage III melanoma

Number of metastatic nodes	Survival rates after node dissection				
	1 year	3 years		5 years	10 years
	(a)	(a)	(b)	(a)	(b)
1	81%	58%	65%	45%	40%
2–4	72%	46%	43%	43%	13%
> 4	65%	28%	22%	15%	

Data from (a) Morton et al. (1985) (150 patients); (b) Balch et al. (1985) (200 patients).

Tumour Thickness

Tumour thickness is still of predictive value in Stage III disease (Milton et al. 1980; Balch et al. 1985; Morton et al. 1985; Berdeaux et al. 1989; Day et al. 1981). The survival rate is low for thick tumours but the number of metastatic nodes is also important. The association of multinodal involvement and tumours thicker than 4 mm is the most pejorative scenario; there was no survivor beyond 14 months in Balch et al.'s study. The presence of ulceration has an additional adverse effect (Balch et al. 1985).

Sex

There is a clear corrective value of sex (in favour of women) in univariate analysis. It may (Cascinelli et al. 1980) or may not (Balch et al. 1985; Berdeaux et al. 1989) persist when matched with other factors.

Therapeutic Factors

The extent of node dissection is an important factor although not well documented; no study mentions incomplete node dissection. Inadequate surgery may expose patients to the risks of further nodal recurrence that are very discouraging and of bad prognosis. All excised nodes must be examined for their situation, extent of metastases and capsular invasion.

Cutaneous Regional Metastases

The prognosis of cutaneous regional metastases is similar to that of nodal metastases. The predictive value of the number and location (superficial or subcutaneous) of metastatic nodules and of the association of nodal metastases (IIIa + b) is not clearly established (Singletary et al. 1988).

In conclusion, the prognosis of regional melanoma is closely correlated to follow-up and rapidity of diagnosis and treatment. Such prompt management may improve the chance of cure or prolong survival (Singletary et al. 1988).

Disseminated Melanoma (Stage IV) (Table 8.7)

The mean clinical course of disseminated melanoma is estimated to be 6 months (Balch et al. 1985). This is very short and confirms the widespread scepticism about the usefulness of systemic treatments, but this mean value only partially reflects the reality and survival can in some cases be very long. In addition to its value in analysing therapeutic results, knowledge of the prognostic factors makes it possible to evaluate the anticipated duration of survival and the likelihood of response to treatment; these factors must be taken into consideration in selecting treatment options.

Factors Related to Primary Lesion and Patient

All the characteristics (histopathological and clinical) of early tumours lose their significance in patients with distant metastases. Age intervenes only by way of performance status which has been found to be predictive of survival (Presant et al. 1982). The survival advantage in women disappears, although this is

Table 8.7. Prognostic factors in disseminated melanoma

Parameters	Prognostic significance
Characteristics of primary tumour	
Histological	–
Clinical	–
Sex	–
Age	–
Performance status	+
Remission time prior to Stage IV	±
Number of metastatic sites	+++
Nature of sites	++
Doubling time	+
Accessibility to radical surgery	++
Response to treatment (complete remission)	++

± Not or partially demonstrated.

controversial and some authors attribute a more rapid evolution in men to androgens (Rampen 1980). In practice, only the characteristics of metastases are predictive.

Number of Metastatic Sites

The number of metastatic sites is the most significant factor in univariate and multivariate analysis. Median survival is shortened by 50% with two sites instead of one (4 *vs.* 7 months) and by 50% again with three sites. Only one-third of patients survive one year or more with one metastatic site and none with three (Balch et al. 1985). This parameter should be taken into consideration in the analysis of therapeutic results.

Site of Distant Metastases

The location of metastases is also an important factor. Pulmonary metastases have the longest median survival (11 months), whereas soft tissue metastases rank second. Bony and cerebral metastases are not so rapidly fatal as hepatic metastases.

Certain specific aspects are especially severe because they indicate a massive spread (miliary pulmonary spread for example) but in paucinodular forms, four or five nodules are not demonstrated to be more pejorative than two or three. The same pertains to bilateral location compared to unilateral location, in symmetrical organs (Delaunay et al. 1991).

Length of Remission

Overall remission time has no influence except at the extremes, but the small numbers of cases in the series do not allow firm conclusions. Patients relapsing within 6–12 months after treatment of initial tumour have a slightly shorter survival (Balch et al. 1985; Delaunay et al. 1991; Roses et al. 1991). Late metastases seem less often to be multiple (Delaunay et al. 1991). Initial metastatic melanomas of unknown origin have a similar prognosis to other metastatic forms but in this case remission time is not known.

Rate of Growth, Doubling Time

Initial rapidity of growth seems to augur a constant and unremitting evolution. Some authors consider that doubling of the dimensions of metastatic nodules within 40 days excludes the possibility of successful surgical excision.

Therapeutic Factors

Only achievement of complete remission would seem to prolong survival noticeably (Delaunay et al. 1991; Roses et al. 1991). In case of solitary metastasis, the complete remission is better provided by surgery, but this concerns only a low percentage of patients. Surgical excision enables mean survival to be prolonged by 6–12 months and more importantly provides 5%–10% of patients with several years' survival.

The impact of partial response on long-term survival is not clear. In any case, regular appreciation of treatment efficacy is fundamental. Any therapeutic modality must be discontinued if there is no measurable response.

Despite this accuracy in determining prognostic factors, melanoma still retains some of the unpredictability that 20 years ago made it infamous. About 5%–10% of melanomas have an unusual course; the very prolonged or regressive evolution even constitutes one of the characteristics of this tumour. The slowly developing forms themselves obey tendencies (female sex, middle age, intermediary thickness, location in extremities) but in reality the unexpected may occur in any type of melanoma and in any context.

In practice, it must be underlined that the prognosis depends on the medical approach: thickness (early diagnosis), number of metastatic nodes in Stage III (follow-up) and at all stages the quality of the therapy (adequacies of excision, thoroughness of node dissection, resection of metastases in cases selected according to precise criteria and evaluation of therapeutic response).

The improvement in prognosis in countries with a high incidence (with the curious result, that the higher the incidence, the better the prognosis) leads to two conclusions: one is optimistic, namely that screening policies and early detection have an impact on overall survival. The other is pessimistic; namely that improvement so far has not been due to any therapeutic progress (Taylor et al. 1984).

References

Ackerman AB (1982) Disagreements about classification of malignant melanomas. Am J Dermatopathol 29:705–726

Balch CM, Milton G (1985) Cutaneous melanoma. Lippincott Philadelphia

Balch CM, Soong S, Murad T, Ingalls A, Halpern N, Maddox W (1979). A multifactorial analysis of melanoma II. Prognostic factors in patients with Stage I melanoma. Surgery 86:343–351

Balch CM, Wilkerson J, Murad T, Soong S, Ingalls A, Maddox W (1980) The prognostic significance of ulceration of cutaneous melanoma. Cancer 45:3012–3017

Balch CM, Soong S, Shaw H, Milton G (1985) An analysis of prognostic factors in 4000 patients with cutaneous melanoma. In: Balch C, Milton G (eds) Cutaneous melanoma. Lippincott, Philadelphia, p 321

Berdeaux D, Meyskens F, Parks B et al. (1989) Cutaneous malignant melanoma. The natural history and prognostic factors influencing the development of Stage II disease. Cancer 63:1430–1436

Blois M, Sagebiel R, Abarbanel R et al. (1983a) Malignant melanoma of the skin. The association of tumor depth and type, and patient sex, age, and site with survival. Cancer 52:1330–1341

Blois M, Sagebiel R, Tuttle M, Caldwell T, Taylor H (1983b) Judging prognosis in malignant melanoma of the skin. Ann Surg 198:83–88

Braun-Falco O, Landthaler M, Holzel D, Konz B, Schmoeckel C (1986) Therapie und Prognose maligner Melanome der Haut. Dtsch Med Wschr 111:1750–1756

Cascinelli N, Morabito A, Bufalino R et al. (WHO collaborating centres for evaluation of methods of diagnosis and treatment of melanoma) (1980) Prognosis of Stage I melanoma of the skin. Int J Cancer 26:733–739

Cassileth B, Lusk E, Tenaglia A (1982) A psychological comparison of patients with melanoma and other dermatologic disorders. J Am Acad Dermatol 7:742–746

Clark W, Elder D, Guerry D et al. (1989) Model prediction survival in Stage I melanoma based on tumor progression. J Natl Cancer Inst 81:1893–1904

Cox EB, Vollmer RT, Seigler HF (1985) Melanoma in the southeastern United States: experience at the Duke Medical Center. In: Balch CM, Milton G (eds.) Cutaneous melanoma. Lippincott, Philadelphia, pp 401–418

Day C, Sober A, Lew R et al. (1981) Malignant melanoma with positive nodes and relatively good prognosis. Cancer 47:955–962

Day C, Mihm M, Sober et al. (1982a) Prognostic factors for melanoma patients with lesions 0.76–1.69 mm in thickness. Ann Surg 195:44–49

Day C, Mihm M, Sober A et al. (1982b) Prognostic factors for patients with clinical Stage I melanoma of intermediate thickness (1.51–3.99 mm). Ann Surg 195:35–43

Day C, Mihm M, Sober A et al. (1982c) A multivariate analysis of prognostic factors for melanoma patients with lesions >3.65 mm in thickness. Ann Surg 195:44–49

Day C, Mihm M, Sober A et al. (1983) Predictors of late deaths among patients with clinical Stage I melanoma who have not had bony or visceral metastases within the first 5 years after diagnosis. J Am Acad Dermatol 8:864–868

Delaunay MM, Amici JH, Avril MF et al. (1991) Chirurgie des metastases pulmonaires et critères d'operabilité. Ann Dermatol Venereol 118:287–295

Drzewiecki K, Andersen K (1982) Survival with malignant melanoma. A regression analysis of prognostic factors. Cancer 49:2414–2419

Drzewiecki K, Frydman H, Andersen K et al. (1990) Malignant melanoma. Changing trends in factors influencing metastasis-free survival from 1964 to 1982. Cancer 65:362–366

Elias E, Didolkar M, Goel I et al. (1977) A clinicopathologic study of prognostic factors in cutaneous malignant melanoma. Surg Gyn Obstet 144:327–333

Funasaka Y, Mishima Y, Ichibashi M et al. (1988) Comparative analysis of oncogene expression and chromosome abnormalities between metastatic and non metastatic B 16 melanoma clones. Dermatologica 177:200–211

Griffel M (1981) Survival of cutaneous malignant melanoma patients at University of Iowa hospitals: 1950–1974. Cancer 47:176–183

Griffiths R, Briggs J (1984) Long term follow-up in cutaneous malignant melanoma: the relationship of maximal tumour thickness to disease free survival, disease recurrence and death. Br J Plastic Surg 37:507–513

Gupta B, Piedmonte M, Karakousis C (1991) Attributes and survival patterns of multiple primary cutaneous malignant melanoma. Cancer 67:1984–1989

Gutman M, Klausner J, Inbar M, Rozin R (1989) Late recurrence of Stage I malignant melanoma. J Surg Oncol 42:96–98

Johnson K, Emrich L, Karakousis C et al. (1985) Comparison of prognostic factors for survival and recurrence in malignant melanoma of the skin. Clinical Stage I. Cancer 55:1107–1117

Karakousis C, Emrich L, Rao U (1989) Tumor thickness and prognosis in clinical Stage I malignant melanoma. Cancer 64:1432

Karjalainen S, Hakulinen T (1988) Survival and prognostic factors of patients with skin melanoma. Cancer 62:2274–2280

Kelly J, Blois M, Sagebiel R (1985a) Frequency and duration of patient follow up after treatment of a primary malignant melanoma. Cancer 56:2287–2291

Kelly J, Sagebiel R, Clyman S, Blois M (1985b) The thin level IV malignant melanoma. Ann Surg 202:98–103

Kopf A, Gross D, Rogers G et al. (1987a) Prognostic index for malignant melanoma. Cancer 59:1236–1241

Kopf AW, Welkovitch B, Frankel RE et al. (1987b) Thickness of malignant melanoma: global analysis of related factors. J Dermatol Surg Oncol 13:345–420

Krementz ET, Reed RJ, Coleman WP et al. (1982) Acral lentiginous melanoma: a clinicopathologic entity. Ann Surg 5:632–645

Kuehnl-Petzoldt C, Wiebelt H, Berger H (1983) Prognostic groups of patients with Stage I melanoma. Arch Dermatol 119:816–819

Lee YT (1980) Diagnosis treatment and prognosis of early melanoma. The importance of depth of micro-invasion. Ann Surg 19:87–97

Lemish W, Heenan J, Holman J et al. (1981) Survival from preinvasive and invasive malignant melanoma in Western Australia. Cancer 52:580–585

Levy E, Silverman M, Vossaert K et al. (1991) Late recurrence of malignant melanoma: a report of five cases, a review of the literature and a study of associated factors. Melanoma Res 1:63–67

MacKie R, Bufalino R, Morabito R et al. (1991) Lack of effect of pregnancy on outcome of melanoma. Cancer 337:653–655

Maize J (1983) Primary cutaneous malignant melanoma. An analysis of the prognostic value of histologic characteristics. J Am Acad Dermatol 8:857–863

McGovern V, Shaw H, Milton G (1983) Prognosis in patients with thin malignant melanoma: influence of regression. Histopathology 7:673–680

Meyskens F, Berdeaux D, Parks B et al. (1988) Cutaneous malignant melanoma. Natural history and prognostic factors influencing survival in patients with Stage I disease. Cancer 62:1207–1214

Milton G, Shaw H, Farago G, MacCarthy W (1980) Tumor thickness and the site and time of first recurrence in cutaneous malignant melanoma. Br J Surg 67:543

Morton D, Roe D, Cochran A (1985) Melanoma in the western United States. In: Balch C, Milton G, (eds) Cutaneous melanoma. Lippincott, Philadelphia

O'Doherty C, Prescott R, White H et al. (1986) Sex differences in presentation and survival from Stage I disease. Cancer 58:788–792

Palangie A, Lassau F, Moreau T, Noury-Duperrat G, Cottenot F (1981) Mélanomes malins de stade I. Importance pronostique de l'épaisseur et du niveau. Nouv Presse Med 10:2337–2340

Pierard E (1988) Do we have markers of the metastatic potential of malignant melanomas. Dermatologica 177:197–199

Podratz KC, Gaffey TA, Symmonds RE et al. (1983) Melanoma of the vulva: an update. Gynecol Oncol 16:153–168

Presant C, Bartolucci A and the Southeastern Cancer Study Group (1982) Prognostic factors in metastatic malignant melanoma. Cancer 49:2192–2196

Rampen FH, Mulder JH (1980) Malignant melanoma: an androgen dependent tumour? Lancet i:562–564

Rogentine G, van Kammen P, Fox B et al. (1979) Psychological factors in the prognosis of malignant melanoma: a prospective study. Psychosomat Med 41:647–655

Rogers G, Kopf A, Rigel D et al. (1983) Effect of anatomical location on prognosis in patients with clinical Stage I melanoma. Arch Dermatol 119:644–649

Rogers G, Kopf A, Rigel D et al. (1986) Hazard-rate analysis in Stage I malignant melanoma. Arch Dermatol 122:999–1002

Ronan SG, Eng AM, Briele HA et al. (1987) Thin malignant melanoma with regression and metastasis. Arch Dermatol 123:1326–1330

Roses D, Karp N, Oratz R et al. (1991) Survival with regional and distant metastases from cutaneous malignant melanoma. Surg Gynecol Obstet 172:262–268

Schmoeckel C, Bockelbrink A, Bockelbrink H et al. (1983) Low- and high-risk malignant melanoma – I Evaluation of clinical and histological prognosticators in 585 cases, Eur J Cancer Clin Oncol 19:227–235

Shaw H, McGovern V, Milton G, Farago G, McCarthy W (1980a) Histologic features of tumors and the female superiority in survival from malignant melanoma. Cancer 45:1604–1608

Shaw H, McGovern V, Milton G et al. (1980b) Malignant melanoma: influence of site of lesion and age of patients in the female superiority in survival. Cancer 46:2731–2735

Shaw H, Milton G (1981) Smoking and the development of metastases from malignant melanoma. Int J Cancer 28:153–156

Shaw H, McCarthy S, McCarthy W, Thompson J, Milton G (1989) Thin regressing malignant melanoma: significance of concurrent regional lymph node metastases. Histopathology 15:257–265

Singletary E, Tucker S, Boddie A (1988) Multivariate analysis of prognostic factors in regional cutaneous metastases of extremity melanoma. Cancer 61:1437–1440

Slingluff CJ, Vollmer RJ, Reingen DS, Seigler HF (1988) Lethal thin malignant melanoma. Ann Surg 208:150–161

Sober A (1989) Cutaneous melanoma in Japan and the United States: comparative prognostic factors. J Invest Dermatol 92:227s–230s

Sober A, Day C, Fitzpatrick T et al. (1983a) Early death from clinical Stage I melanoma. J Invest Dermatol 80:050s–052s

Sober A, Day C, Fitzpatrick T et al. (1983b) Factors associated with death from melanoma from 2 to 5 years following diagnosis in clinical Stage I patients. J Invest Dermatol 80:53s–55s

Sondergaard K, Olsen G (1980) Malignant melanoma of the foot. A clinicopathological study of 125 primary cutaneous malignant melanomas. Acta Pathol Microbiol Immunol Scand (A) 88:275–283

Soong S (1985) Cutaneous melanoma. A computerized mathematical model and scoring system for predicting outcome in melanoma patients. In: Balch CM, Milton G (eds.) Cutaneous melanoma. Lippincott, Philadelphia, pp 353–370

Stolz W, Schmoeckel C, Welkovich B, Braun-Falco O (1989) Semiquantitative analysis of histologic criteria in thin malignant melanomas. Acad Dermatol 20:1115–1120

Taylor B, Hughes L, Williams G (1984) Improving prognosis for malignant melanoma in Britain. Br J Surg 71:950–953

Temoshek L, Heller B, Sagebiel R et al. (1985) The relationship of psychosocial factors to prognostic indicators in cutaneous malignant melanoma. J Psychosom Res 29:139–153

Tonak J, Hermanek P, Weidner F, Geggenmoos-Holzmann I, Altendorf A (1985) Melanoma in Germany: experience at the University of Erlangen-Nuremburg. In: Balch CM, Milton G (eds.) Cutaneous melanoma. Lippincott, Philadelphia, pp 483–494

Trau H, Rigel Harris H et al. (1983) Metastases of thin melanomas. Cancer 51:553–556

van der Esch E, Cascinelli N, Preda F et al. (1981) Stage I melanoma: evaluation of prognosis according to histologic characteristics. Cancer 48:1668–1673

Watzig V, Knopf B (1981) Combination of high risk factors as an accurate guide to prognosis in malignant melanoma. Eur J Cancer Clin Oncol 17:1237–1240

Weidner F (1981) Eight years survival in malignant melanoma related to sex and tumor location. Dermatologica 162:51–60

Worth A, Gallagher R, Elwood J et al. (1989) Pathologic prognostic factors for cutaneous malignant melanoma: the western Canada melanoma study. Int J Cancer 43:370–375

9   Surgery for Malignant Melanoma

Judy Evans

The treatment of malignant melanoma remains largely surgical. However, the last decade has seen a major swing away from indiscriminate radical surgery. The development of prognostic indicators, and a more scientific approach to surgery has meant that a better informed public, presenting with early disease, can be offered less radical, safe surgery, that can be cosmetically more acceptable.

Surgery of nodal disease has been refined, and on occasion combined with regional chemotherapy. Isolated non-nodal metastases may be surgically removed. Long-term disease-free survival is not uncommon following such procedures.

Finally, surgery may be important in achieving good palliation. This is probably the only area in melanoma treatment where surgery has become more aggressive in recent years.

Surgeons and their nursing teams are likely to be the most constant attendants to melanoma patients. They may be involved with treatment and follow-up over many years. The importance of developing a good relationship with the patient can never be overstated. However, early introduction of the patient to a multidisciplinary team may be very valuable, if the patient progresses to advanced disease. The surgeon must ensure patients are well informed, appropriately reassured and educated in self-examination. Surgery can therefore be considered in four phases of melanoma treatment:

1. Diagnostic
2. Definitive primary treatment
3. Surgery of nodal metastases, and other potentially curable metastatic sites
4. Palliative surgery

Diagnostic Surgery

There is no place for incisional biopsy to gain a diagnosis of melanoma. A biopsy should be a whole tumour, full skin thickness biopsy with a 2 mm clear margin around the entire tumour, with a cuff of subdermal fat.

Historically, controversy raged about the safety of incisional biopsy, with some publications suggesting this technique disseminated malignant cells and others demonstrating that it did not. The modern objection to incisional biopsy is that it is no longer sufficient to demonstrate that a tumour is a melanoma. A tumour must be histologically staged both in terms of its absolute maximum thickness (Breslow) and in its penetration through the layers of the skin (Clark's levels). An incisional biopsy cannot guarantee to sample the maximum tumour thickness, and a subsequent whole tumour biopsy may be altered by postsurgical inflammation so that an accurate tumour thickness cannot be obtained.

In Britain public awareness of the dangers of leaving pigmented lesions is increasing, and the majority of patients present with small early lesions. There remains a significant minority who have not heard of, or deliberately choose to ignore the dangers associated with "changing moles".

Biopsy Technique

Local anaesthetic is routinely used, except in small children or patients who will not tolerate a local anaesthetic procedure.

There is a theoretical risk that the administration of local anaesthetic into a lesion will increase the tissue turgor to such an extent that tumour cells will detach and disseminate. This would be difficult to demonstrate and is as yet unproven. This risk can be avoided by the insertion of local anaesthetic circumferentially around the lesion, a small distance from its periphery.

It is the author's preference to close biopsy wounds wherever possible, except where a local flap, or graft is required to achieve closure. In these cases a circular wound may be left open with a moisture-retaining dressing until definitive histology is obtained. Only then will available local tissue be transposed into a wound, if appropriate.

The technique of biopsy should be explained to the patient, who should then be asked to lie on a couch, or operating table. The provision of good lighting is essential, so that the edges of a tumour may be clearly seen. The skin surrounding the lesion should be cleansed, the area dried, and the edge of the tumour marked with Bonney's Blue. This may seem a superfluous step with a uniformly pigmented lesion, but it is particularly important to outline the extent of the tumour where there is peripheral regression or depigmentation. Once the lesion is fully defined, attention is turned to the most appropriate method of closing the wound. The skin in the immediate area should be pinched between finger and thumb, in two directions, perpendicular to each other. In this way the direction of least tissue tension can be established, and an appropriate ellipse mapped out (Fig. 9.1). The minimum clearance is always measured as 2 mm.

Local anaesthetic is then inserted around the periphery of the marked ellipse. The author uses 2% lignocaine with adrenaline 1:80 000, using a dental syringe. This local anaesthetic is almost immediately effective. The skin is incised with a vertical cut through the whole thickness of the skin. A keel-shaped portion of subdermal fat is included with the lesion. Bipolar diathermy is used to coagulate small subdermal vessels where necessary, and the wound closed with interrupted monofilament nylon sutures of appropriate thickness. Deep sutures are avoided wherever possible. The vertical cut through the skin edges lends itself to good apposition. A light dressing is applied to cover the wound, and the patient given

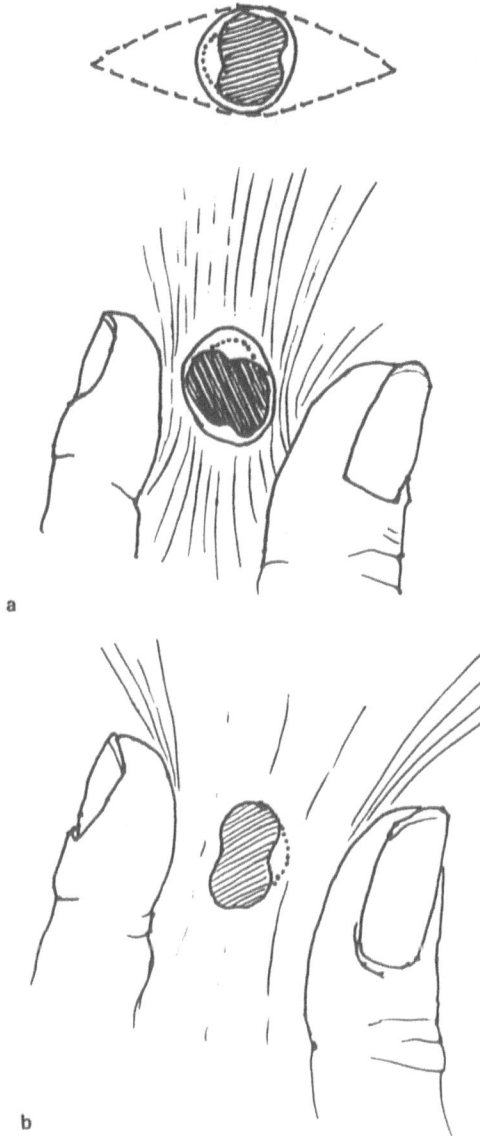

Fig. 9.1. To show ellipse. **a** Incorrect direction; **b** correct direction with least tissue tension and appropriate skin ellipse.

an early appointment to return to discuss the histology report and any further treatment.

In the author's practice, an increasing number of patients request biopsy of lesions which have shown recent change, but which are not clinically suggestive of melanoma. Such patients are very reassured by a diagnosis of a benign lesion and a neat, small scar. It is always desirable to achieve a cosmetically acceptable scar after biopsy, even when patients have to go on to further excision. Patients may gain confidence from this exhibit of the surgeon's ability to produce neat wounds.

Histology Reporting

The demands on the histopathologist are high. He or she must be able to state that the lesion is a malignant melanoma. Doubtful reports are returned with a request for special stains or referral to a specialist in melanoma histopathology. All reports should include a Breslow thickness measurement, a Clark's level, describe intravascular invasion, ulceration where present, and comment on the mitotic index.

The author regards the Breslow thickness as the most important prognostic indicator, and uses Clark's level as a modifier. In this way thin lesions that arise in thin skin, and are already extending throughout the dermis will be picked up. Ulceration, regression and the presence of pre-existing benign naevi may make the Breslow thickness difficult to measure, this must be borne in mind when considering this measurement. There is still debate as to the role of frozen section specimens in the diagnosis and staging of melanomas. The author does not request this and prefers to wait for paraffin section, which can be available within 24 hours.

Definitive Primary Treatment

This depends on the biopsy report. This author places the tumour into one of three risk groups (Bagley et al. 1981).

Low risk: less than 0.76 mm thick, Clark's level II or III

Medium risk: less than 0.76 mm thick, Clark's level IV. All tumours between 0.76 and 1.5 mm

High risk: greater than 1.5 mm thick, Clark's level IV. All Clark's level V

Definitive treatment is then prescribed according to risk group as follows:

Risk group	Clearance margin
Low	2 mm (i.e. biopsy)
Medium	20 mm
High	50 mm

Anatomical sites where such excisions are not possible, e.g. face, scalp, digits, anal margin, are treated as special cases and the details of their surgery meticulously recorded.

Preliminary results show that this approach to the treatment of malignant melanoma is safe (Table 9.1).

Table 9.1. Recurrences after definitive primary treatment

Risk group (total no. of patients in group)	Local no. (%) of patients	Nodal no. (%) of patients
Low ($n = 0$)	0(0)	0(0)
Median ($n = 5$)	0(0)	5(3)
High ($n = 107$)	39(10)	68(17)

Other Protocols Described for Definitive Treatment to Malignant Melanoma

Taylor et al. (1984) have proposed a protocol where the minimum excision margin is 1 cm around the tumour, for lesions up to 1 mm thick, and a further 1 cm clearance, up to a total of 3 cm radius for every millimetre of tumour thickness.

Veronesi et al. (1988) in a World Health Organization multicentre trial proposed either a 1 cm or 3 cm margin of excision. Out of 305 patients with a 1 cm excision, only three had a local recurrence as a first relapse, these three all had primary tumours of 1 mm or more thick.

At the time of writing, there is a widespread trend away from radical excisions for all lesions, regardless of histological prognostic factors. All the protocols described above require a further long period of follow-up before final answers to the question of resection margin size will be found.

Techniques of Definitive Primary Treatment

In the simplest lesions the excisions may be closed directly, as previously described for the biopsy. Where it is not possible to close a small wound by means of a simple ellipse, local flaps, either sliding, rotation or transposition flaps may be used to avoid having to perform a graft. These are well described in basic textbooks of plastic surgery (MacGregor 1989).

In the large excisions, closure of wounds with split skin grafts remain the mainstay of treatment. Modern techniques of wound closure attempt to reduce the size of these defects, and to minimize the contour defects created by excision of skin and fat down to deep fascia. Tissue expansion techniques, and serial excisions of split skin grafts, may, by a series of cosmetic operations after definitive surgery, totally eliminate contour deficiencies in time.

Technique of Wide Excision and Grafting

These operations are usually performed under general anaesthetic. The patient is prepared for surgery in the normal way. The biopsy site is marked and a skin graft donor site discussed with the patient, and agreed preoperatively. The (non-involved) thigh is the commonest donor site, the inner aspect of the arm may be used in some patients, especially where early mobilization is preferred, because of other medical conditions.

The operative fields are cleaned and the patient towelled. The extent of the excision is measured around the biopsy site, and marked out as a circle. It is good practice in these cases to harvest the skin for grafting before operating on the biopsy site. The donor site can thus be dressed before there is any surgical contact with the biopsy site. The donor area may be very painful postoperatively. The author routinely injects bupivicaine 0.25% subdermally under the donor site prior to graft harvest in an attempt to reduce postoperative pain. Partial thickness skin is then taken with a skin grafting knife. The author aims to take sufficient skin to cover the defect completely, plus approximately one-third of this area again, as spare skin, to be used in the event of graft failure. The donor site wound is then dressed completely. The definitive excision consists of removal of skin and underlying fat, down to, but not including deep fascia. The surgery proceeds as for the initial biopsy, with a vertical, full thickness cut through the skin. Excision of slightly more fat than skin, with the creation of an "upside down saucer" defect follows. This allows the skin edges to be approximated to underlying fascia in such a way as to minimize the contour defect, and eliminate an ugly 'Cliff' effect which remains if fat and skin are cut vertically (Fig. 9.2). It is important to clear the fat cleanly from underlying deep fascia in order to get a good take of graft, and a smooth appearance. The size of the defect can be reduced somewhat by suturing the skin down to fascia, under slight tension. The graft is then placed on the remaining exposed fascia, and either sutured, or stapled in place. A firm pressure dressing is then applied and left for 48 hours. In some sites it may be necessary to use a tie-over dressing to apply uniform pressure and prevent haematoma formation floating the graft off the base of the wound.

A single sheet of good quality skin graft is likely to give the best cosmetic result from a grafting operation. However, where cosmetic considerations are of low priority, or where poor healing is anticipated, meshing the graft prior to application may improve, or accelerate, graft take.

After initial inspection of the graft at 48 hours, further firm dressings may be applied for, on average, another ten days. Once the skin is fully healed, the patient should be advised to wear a pressure or support stocking in limb lesions. This is to prevent or minimize any lymphoedema caused by surgical division of local lymphatics.

In a series of 100 consecutive patients requiring skin grafts to the lower leg, average hospital stay was 12 days (Plymouth, unpublished data). Patients in low-risk groups who can receive definitive treatment without hospitalization are saved this prolonged stay and its attendant psychological and social trauma.

Once the wounds are healed, frequent follow-up is required to detect local or distance recurrences, and also to teach the patient self-examination. The importance of self-examination and the recognition by the patient of easy access

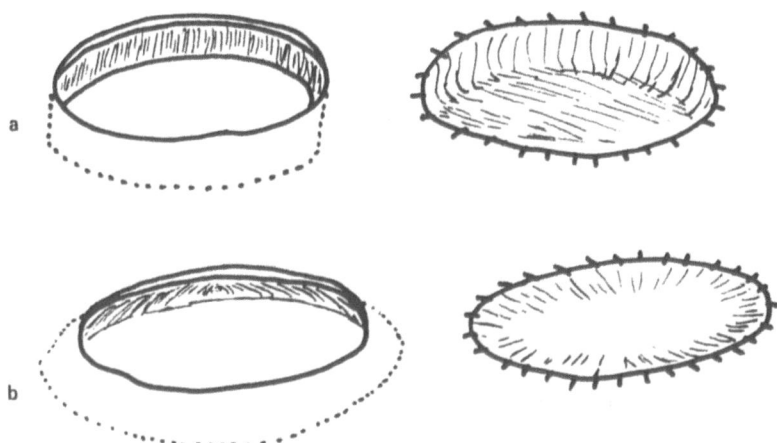

Fig. 9.2. Excision of skin: **a** with vertical cut through fat, leading to "cliff effect"; **b** with undercutting of fat leading to flattened smoothed edge.

to the surgical team is repeated at each visit. Follow-up is initially monthly with increasing intervals, up to five years, with a once yearly appointment after that time.

Later Aesthetic Plastic Surgery

Patients vary very considerably in their self-consciousness of the external appearance of the surgical defect. Some patients accept the advice that it is best to wait for five years free of recurrence before considering cosmetic reconstruction. Others may hide away and alter their lifestyles very drastically because of an inability to come to terms with the defect. In these cases there should be no hard and fast rule about the timing of aesthetic reconstruction. Careful counselling and support from the surgeon may be helpful, but there are cases where early reconstruction has been mandatory because of the patient's suicidal attitude to the deformity. Close liaison with a clinical psychologist attached to the surgical team has proved very helpful in identifying and treating such patients.

Aesthetic plastic surgery to grafted areas involves replacing an area where skin graft is lying on fascia with full thickness soft tissue, appropriate to the local area. This can be achieved by:

1. *Multiple excision* of the centre of the grafted area (the technique of serial excision) until the graft is completely removed
2. *Use of a tissue expander* which is a silastic balloon with a filler device that can be inserted under normal soft tissue adjacent to the graft. Over a period of approximately three months, this is filled with saline, and the overlying tissue expanded. Finally the expander is removed, and the expanded tissue used to replace the skin graft
3. In certain cases a local flap, without expansion, may be rotated into the defect to eliminate the contour defect of the graft.

Curative Surgery for Metastases

At present the author does not practise elective regional node dissection, or in-continuity block dissection. There is, as yet, no convincing evidence that such a procedure produces benefit to the majority of patients, although some studies have shown an increase in disease-free interval in a narrowly defined group of patients. The author believes that free access to the unit and frequent follow-up allow early detection of clinically involved lymph nodes. Major trials are currently in progress to elucidate the role of nodal dissection, and also concomitant perfusion of isolated limbs with chemotherapeutic agents.

The commonest sites for nodal metastases are the axillary glands, the cervical glands and the inguinal glands. These are treated by standard block dissection techniques as described in many excellent textbooks of operative surgery. Special features will be briefly discussed. There are occasions when there is doubt about the nature of enlarged glands, particularly for example, if a grafted primary lesion has become infected. The use of fine needle aspiration biopsy has been found to be very helpful in such cases, although false negatives do occur.

Inguinal Node Dissection

Where a nodal mass is close to the skin, an ellipse of skin is included in the block dissection specimen and sacrificed. One of the most common complications of this operation is delayed healing and skin loss at the mid-point of the scar. This modification seems to reduce the frequency of such skin loss.

The author normally performs a sub (inguinal) ligamentous dissection with sampling of Cloquet's node. There is no evidence to suggest that combined inguinal and para-aortic node dissection is of benefit and the further dissection contributes to increased morbidity.

Transposition of the sartorius muscle, detaching it from its origin, and rotating it around its long axis medially to cover the femoral vessels, is considered essential.

Inguinal block dissection wounds are always drained, using a vacuum drainage system. Patient mobilization may be delayed by prolonged drainage of lymph like fluid from these drains. It is the author's impression that this can be minimized by paying particular attention to haemostasis of any minor oozing from the most distal part of the dissection.

Post-operatively the patients' most frequent complaints are of lymphoedema. All patients should be warned in advance of the likelihood of this problem, and early conservative management should be instituted where appropriate to relieve symptoms, e.g. compression stockings, periodic elevation and bed rest and 'Flowtron boots'.

Axillary Block Dissection

Several incisions are described for axillary block dissection, of which the author favours a longitudinal mid-axillary incision, from the upper arm down on to the chest wall. This operation varies slightly according to the site of the primary lesion. Greater attention is paid to subdermal lymphatics in the arm where a limb primary is involved. Radical clearance of all tissue around the axillary vessels is meticulously performed.

Excellent access to the apex of the axilla may be achieved by detaching the origin of the pectoralis minor muscle. This gives a very clear view of even a very obese axilla. There is a slightly increased morbidity because of this manoeuvre; occasional cases of rupture of the muscle repair, or intramuscular haematoma have necessitated re-exploration.

The wounds are routinely drained, with suction drainage which has an important role in closing dead space, and promoting good apposition of flaps.

Cervical Block Dissection

The author does not favour elective node dissection, and therefore does not perform functional neck dissections in the presence of established metastatic disease. The axillary nerve, sternomastoid muscle and internal jugular vein are all sacrificed. The patient must be fully warned preoperatively of the likely deformity and difficulty with shoulder movement. On occasion this operation is combined with a total parotidectomy; the facial paralysis resulting from such surgery must also be carefully explained to the patient.

A champagne glass incision is preferred; the flaps are dissected at the subplatysmal level. Any potentially involved skin is again excised with the main tissue block. Local flaps or flaps from the chest wall may need to be introduced if there is extensive skin involvement.

In cases of posterior primary lesions, from the angle of mandible, or in the region of the ear, zone I (the submental area) is left intact where there is no evidence of antegrade spread. There is little evidence to suggest perineural spread in melanoma, nerve sampling does not form a prominent feature of this operation.

Wounds are routinely drained with suction drains to ensure close apposition and good survival of skin flaps. If patients become confused following neck dissection and there is evidence of swelling at the operative site, early re-exploration in theatre may be life saving. Haematoma formation causing external compression of the trachea is an occasional complication.

In all block dissections, after haemostasis the author irrigates the wound with warm water. Mechanical cleansing and the administration of a hypotonic solution may have a role in reducing tumour seeding.

Curative Surgery to Other Metastases

Occasional isolated metastases may be found on scanning. Single intracranial lesions are occasionally seen, and should be treated by radical excision, involving a full craniotomy if necessary.

Single local recurrences close to the primary site should be treated by excision and grafting. When such a lesion occurs close to a limb primary, the patient should be considered for isolated limb perfusion.

Once it has become obvious that a single recurrence is only the first sign of widespread disease, the emphasis should change to palliation.

Palliative Surgery

Widespread subdermal nodules may be the first evidence of overwhelming disseminated disease. Such patients should be considered for treatment with chemotherapy or biological response modifiers. There is still a place for surgery when particular lesions become troublesome.

Patients are generally offered the choice of which, if any, of these lesions should be removed. Reasons for opting for surgery include:

Large size of individual nodule

Potential or actual ulceration of nodule, or infection

Painful nodule

Nodule interferes with function, or wearing of clothes

Patient requests removal because appearance of nodule causes distress

Inability to sleep because of pain in lying position

Patient wishes the surgeon to continue to remove as much tumour as possible

Deep seated metastases may cause severe symptoms early in their growth. An example of this is intussusception and consequent obstruction caused by intraluminal intestinal metastases. A laparotomy with a partial bowel resection may be very worthwhile in such cases, returning the patients to a relative state of good health, and able to eat and drink again, even if only for a few months.

At this last stage of a patient's disease, a very close liaison between surgical teams, oncologists, radiotherapists, psychologists and social workers is very helpful. Specialist surgeons such as neurosurgeons and urologists may also need to be closely involved. Although the medical attendants must make the ultimate assessment of the worth of major treatments in the patient's last few months, it is at this stage of the disease more than any other that the patient must have greatest influence on the extent of treatment.

References

Bagley FH, Cady B, Lee A, Legg MA (1981) Changes in clinical presentation and management of malignant melanoma. Cancer 47:2126–2134

MacGregor IA (1989) Fundamental techniques of plastic surgery and their applications, 8th edn. Churchill Livingstone, Edinburgh

Taylor BA, Hughes LE, Williams GT (1984) Improving prognosis for malignant melanoma in Britain. Br J Surg 71:950–953

Veronesi U, Cascinelli N, Adumus J et al. (1988) Thin Stage I primary cutaneous malignant melanoma. Comparison of excision with margins of 1 or 3 cm. N Engl J Med 318:1159–1162

10 Isolated Limb Perfusion

R. D. Rosin

The principal of regional perfusion using cytostatic drugs resulted from a study by Klopp et al. (1950) who found that pain was alleviated and tumour size reduced when small doses of nitrogen mustard were injected into the regional arterial blood flow. The best results were obtained when venous return from the area involved was blocked. In 1956, the coming together of a cardiothoracic, a plastic and an oncological surgeon in the Department of Surgery at Tulane University, New Orleans, Louisiana, USA, resulted in the introduction of a new concept in the treatment of regionally recurrent malignant disease. It was postulated that if an area of the body could be isolated from the systemic circulation and sustained by an extracorporeal circuit utilizing a heart lung machine, it would be possible to produce a high concentration of a chemotherapeutic agent in the isolated perfusion circuit limited only by the toxicity to the sensitive structures within that area. At the end of the perfusion, the unbound drug could be removed, the circulation restored and any excisional surgery carried out as necessary. The patient would benefit by a maximal tumour chemotherapeutic exposure in the treated area while being protected from systemic toxicity. Ryan et al. (1957) developed techniques in the laboratory for isolation perfusion of the hind limb, mid gut and liver of a dog. It was found that the dosage of nitrogen mustard tolerated in the hind limb was the equivalent of a single whole body systemic dose.

In 1957, a 76-year-old man presented with recurrent melanoma of the left lower limb consisting of more than 80 cutaneous satellites following a previous wide excision of a melanoma of the ankle and superficial groin dissection in 1955. Perfusion of the left lower leg was carried out with a home made, De Wall-type bubble oxygenator and a Sigma motor pump (Creech et al. 1959). Melphalan (120 mg) was used in the circuit and over the period of the next several months, a gradual remission of the satellites occurred. Total clearing of the recurrent melanoma followed. The patient survived 16 years, dying free of disease aged 92. This unique response stimulated the development of the clinical use of isolated perfusion with chemotherapy for recurrent regional malignancy.

Technique of Isolated Limb Perfusion

Upper Limb Perfusion (Fig. 10.1)

An incision is made in the subclavicular region. The clavicular and sternal portions of the pectoralis major are separated and the pectoralis minor is detached from the coracoid process. This exposes the intermediate and superior levels of the axilla. The latter are radically dissected and all collateral vessels are ligated. The patient is then fully heparinized following which first the axillary vein and then the artery are cannulated. An Esmarch's bandage is then tightened around the shoulder, anchored with Steinman pins inserted into the subcutaneous tissue around the root of the limb. After one hour perfusion, and subsequent washout of the vasculature with approximately 2 litres of Hartmann's solution, the tourniquet is removed, the cannulas are taken out of first the artery and then the vein and the arteriotomy and then the venotomy are repaired with continuous Prolene sutures.

A full axillary block dissection is performed as it is extremely difficult to assess this region following isolated limb perfusion. Perfusion is carried out for recurrent disease usually with three drugs: melphalan, actinomycin D and nitrogen mustard. If a repeat perfusion is being performed then vindesine or DTIC are used.

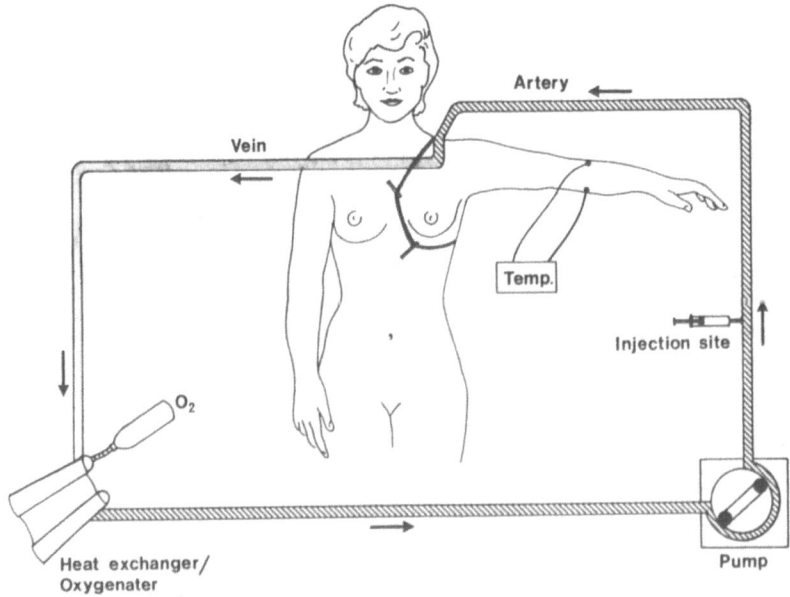

Fig. 10.1. Upper extremity isolated limb perfusion. Reproduced from Rosin (1991), with permission.

Lower Limb Perfusion (Fig. 10.2)

A skin crease incision is made in the iliac fossa and the external iliac vessels are approached extraperitoneally. An ilio-obturator lymph node clearance is performed up to the bifurcation of the common iliac artery. All collateral vessels situated behind the inguinal ligament are controlled and/or divided following which the patient is heparinized. The internal iliac artery and vein are then cross clamped. The external iliac vein is cannulated followed by cannulation of the external iliac artery as for an upper limb perfusion. A Steinman pin is inserted into the anterior superior iliac spine and a tourniquet made of an Esmarch's bandage strongly tightened around the root of the limb over the Steinman pin.

In older patients who have disease confined to below the knee, a femoral isolated limb perfusion may be performed placing an inflatable tourniquet above the mid-thigh incision. With this type of perfusion, there is rarely any leak at all.

Preparation of the limb to be perfused In the operating theatre Thermistor probes are inserted into the subcutaneous tissue on the distal part of the limb and into the forearm or calf musculature. The limb is then wrapped in silver foil to insulate it.

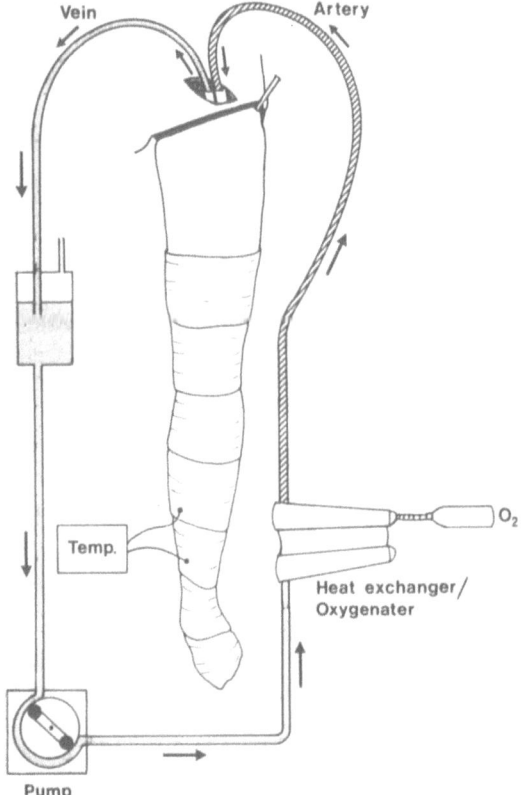

Fig. 10.2. Iliac isolated limb perfusion. Reproduced from Rosin (1991), with permission.

Extracorporeal circulation in isolated perfusion The extracorporeal circuit consists of a roller pump and a membrane oxygenator with 2 cm silicone tubing. The pump is primed with Hartmann's solution and on occasion, the leg is drained to prime the pump. Perfusate flow is set as high as possible, that is with blood levels in the reservoir at equilibrium. Leakage is measured with radioactive albumin which is injected into the circuit and assessed centrally.

The input temperature is kept at 41°C and the drug(s) is given once the skin temperature has reached 40°C, in divided doses at 0, 15 and 30 min. This method is used in case the leak should be too high when the second and/or third dose can be omitted.

Historical

In 1960, Stehlin et al. reported 116 regional perfusions performed at the M.D. Anderson Hospital, Houston. Luck (1956) discovered that melphalan (L-phenylaline mustard) was the most active in inhibiting the growth of malignant melanoma in mice. This has since been the agent of choice in perfusion. In 1967, Cavaliere et al. laid the foundation for perfusions under hyperthermia when they described the susceptibility of cancer cells to high temperatures. Westbury (Rosin and Westbury 1980) in fact had commenced isolated limb perfusion in 1960 and soon after had heated the circuit on the grounds that melphalan worked better at a higher temperature.

Favourable results with regional limb perfusion have been reported by numerous investigators since Creech et al.'s original description in 1959 (Rochlin and Smart 1965; Schraffordt Koops et al. 1977, 1981; Illig and Aigner 1980; Martijn et al. 1981, 1982, 1986; McBride et al. 1981; Aigner et al. 1983; Jonsson et al. 1983; Lejeune et al. 1983; Tonak et al. 1983; Krementz et al. 1985; Storm and Morton 1985; Israels 1987; Lejeune 1987; Vaglini et al. 1987; Franklin et al. 1988; Ghussen et al. 1988; Kroon 1988). Perfusion of melanomas in other parts of the body is not possible because leakage to the systemic circulation could become excessive and the advantage of regional perfusion, that is, high local dosage of the cytostatic agents without systemic toxic reactions, is lost. However, perfusion with ultrafiltration may be possible in these situations.

Indications for Isolated Limb Perfusion

Originally, this modality of treatment was used for in-transit metastases not amenable to surgery on a limb. Over the last 30 years, as it has proved its worth for recurrent disease, attempts have been made to use it to reduce the rate of recurrence and improve survival in high risk clinical stage I patients.

It is now our standard practice to perform therapeutic isolated limb perfusions for local recurrences and in-transit metastases in a limb. Routinely, three drugs are used, melphalan, actinomycin D and nitrogen mustard. For subsequent perfusions, second line therapy such as DTIC or vindesine is used.

Clinical Stage I poor prognosis melanomas on a limb in our institution are also perfused. However, this prophylactic perfusion has not yet been proven to be of benefit in a randomized prospective trial. Indications for prophylactic perfusion and the results to date will be discussed.

The dosages of the chemotherapeutic agents can be calculated on the basis of total body weight but this does not take into account the wide variation in limb volumes that can be found for the same body weight (Vaglini et al. 1983). Other methods for calculating the dosage can be by determining the exact volume of the limb by immersing it in water (Wieberdink et al. 1982). Lejeune and Ghanem (1987) had described a dosimetric method which is based on the exchangeable blood volume determination of the perfused limb. This volume has been calculated by haematocrit measurements of the priming of the peripheral blood before cannulation, and of the mixed perfusate after cannulation.

Complications

A tissue reaction of the extremity is seen approximately 48 h after perfusion. The extremity is usually red, warm and slightly oedematous. The redness fades to brown which gradually over 3–6 months becomes lighter. After approximately six months, there is no visible evidence of any change. Some patients suffer drying and blistering of the palms or soles of the feet and loss of hair occurs. With increased experience and improvement of isolation techniques, bone marrow depression should not occur.

During the period 1980–1990, more than 200 patients have been submitted to isolated limb perfusion. Only one in-hospital death has occurred from cardiac and renal failure.

Deep vein thrombosis can occur and is extremely difficult to diagnose clinically. We now routinely carry out Doppler flow studies in the postoperative period. Oedema with erythema occurs in approximately 15% of patients, but this is usually mild and easily controlled with a graduated compression stocking. Marked persisting oedema occurred in only 2% of the patients. Most of these had had a concurrent deep vein thrombosis. Arterial damage occurred in three patients, an intimal flap being raised in two upper limb perfusions and in one lower limb. There were no cases of retroperitoneal haemorrhage and wound infection only when the lower limb perfusion was carried out via the femoral route together with femoral triangle block dissection.

Systemic complications were rare and were mainly infections of either the urinary or respiratory tract. Thrombogranulopenia was usually secondary to a high leak rate (greater than 10%) after five minutes of perfusion.

Results of Therapeutic Isolated Limb Perfusion

Experience gained from reviewing the perfusions performed at Westminster Hospital from 1960 to 1979 (Rosin and Westbury 1980) and at St Mary's Hospital from 1980 to 1990 confirms the validity of regional treatment of melanoma. A total of 45% of our patients survive for five years but less than 30% were disease free. The majority of recurrences in the limb occurred within two years. Although the staging is different from that used in the M.D. Anderson staging Krementz (1987) gives salvage rates of 60% at 10 years and 46% at 20 years for Stage II disease. For Stage III or regionally recurrent disease, survival rates were 42% at 10 years and 38% at 20 years. Schraffordt Koops et al. (1990) give a five-year disease-free and actual survival for their 110 patients of 35% and 61% respectively. Their five-year disease-free survival for Stage II disease was 58%, for Stage IIIA 27% and for Stage IIIAB 21%. The five-year actuarial survival for Stage II was 74%, for Stage IIIA 67% and for Stage IIIAB 40%. Again, they have used the M.D. Anderson staging. Lejeune et al. (1989) in their 182 patients had a disease-free survival of 27% in Stage II disease and a five-year overall survival of 53.5%. They state that in contrast with their poor disease-free survival, 67% of patients treated with two or more perfusions showed a five-year survival.

Five-year survival rates after perfusion for patients with local recurrences, satellites or in-transit metastases range from 31% to 74% with a tendency to better survival in those patients with "local recurrence" (Table 10.1). According to the EORTC experience (Lejeune et al. 1989) conventional surgery allows disease-free survival in their Stage II patients of 25% and a five-year survival of 30. It must be pointed out that the use of isolated limb perfusion therapeutically has virtually negated the need for amputation. Lejeune et al. have also shown that in their series only 24% developed distant metastases as the first sign of recurrence. They state that this finding further supports a concept of regional treatment with isolated perfusion. In 24 patients who were submitted to further perfusions for new regional recurrences, the disease-free interval was poor being 4% at three years but survival was unexpectedly high, 67% at five years after the first perfusion. They have suggested that repeat perfusions for multiple recurrences of melanoma render the tumour less aggressive although rarely eradicated.

Isolated regional perfusion has been justified by many surgeons for recurrent melanoma of the extremities. Au and Goldman (1977) have pointed out that the disease has already demonstrated aggressive behaviour in those patients with recurrences and these will progress unless the course of the disease can be modified. Even in the most advanced cases, five-year survivals have been given as approximately 35%. Although isolated perfusion with chemotherapeutic agents has been practised for more than 30 years, many questions are yet unanswered. Although it is known that there is an evident enhancement with certain drugs, there are no conclusive data showing an improvement of the therapeutic index of rising temperature. The optimal temperature has not yet been agreed and normothermia (temperature between 37° and 38°C), mild hyperthermia (temperatures held between 39° and 40.5°C) and hyperthermia have all been used in different institutions. In the great majority of series, the temperature is usually in the range of mild hyperthermia. Also although melphalan is a well tried and tested drug, dosages vary and its combination with other drugs has not been standardized. Perhaps different combinations than those already used might improve results. Also the place of repeat perfusions and the combination of perfusion with infusion have not been fully explored. As isolated regional perfusion is a considerable physical and financial burden, as well as having a morbidity, it is a pity that the questions posed have not been answered over the last 30 years.

Table 10.1. Results of regional perfusion in patients with local recurrence (II), in-transit metastases (IIIA) and local recurrence and/or in-transit metastases + positive lymph nodes (IIIAB)

Author	Year	Cytostatics	Number of patients	Local recurrence rate in the perfused limb	5-year survival rate (%)			10/year survival rate (%)		
					II	IIIA	IIIAB	II	IIIA	IIIAB
Krementz et al.	1985	melphalan	182	–	64	35	31	58	28	28
Shiu et al.	1986	nitrogen mustard	18	–	–	50	38	–	–	–
Cavaliere et al.	1987	melphalan	65	–	80	56	33	–	–	–
Hartley and Fletcher	1987	melphalan	39	–	58[a]		29	44[a]		29
Stehlin et al.	1988	melphalan	117	–	75	70	36	–	50	23
Hoekstra et al.	1989	melphalan ± actinomycin D	110	38	74	67	40	63	45	34

[a] Hartley and Fletcher did not discriminate between stage II and IIIA.

Prophylactic Isolated Limb Perfusion

Although most oncologists agree that regional perfusion is an effective treatment for satellitosis or regionally confined melanoma, to date there has been no prospective randomized trial carried out to prove the efficacy of chemotherapy by perfusion as adjuvant therapy for Stage I melanoma. Ghussen et al. (1988) did undertake a prospective randomized trial for melanoma of the limbs with excision and perfusion verses excision alone but it was discontinued after three and a half years as more favourable results were obtained in the group of patients who were subjected to perfusion as well as excision.

Recurrence rates of less than 2% and five-year survival from 70% to 95% have been reported with isolation perfusion in high risk melanoma of the extremities (Table 10.2). However, there is some controversy regarding the effectiveness of prophylactic isolation perfusion, some authors claiming that recurrence and survival rates were similar to the results of conventional surgery.

Table 10.2. Adjuvant isolated limb perfusion for Stage I malignant melanoma

Authors	Date	No. of patients	Control	Randomized	Result
Rochlin and Smart	1965	101	None	No	95% Disease free at 4 years
McBride et al.	1975	202	Historical	No	83% 10 year survival 18% RLN
Davis et al.	1975	72	None	No	90% 5 year survival
Sugarbaker and McBride	1976	199	None	No	83% 5 year survival
Golomb	1976	57	Yes	No	5 year survival 96% vs 84%
Stehlin	1980	70	None	No	83.5% 5 year survival
Schraffordt Koops et al.	1981	132	None	No	78% 5 year survival
Rege et al	1983	30	Yes	No	"Significant" improvement of survival
Ghussen et al.	1984	37	Yes	Yes	Discontinued as highly significant
Krementz	1986	381	No	None	80% 10 year survival
MRC/MSG/BASO	1988–90	36	Yes	Yes	Closed – poor accrual
WHO/EORTC/NAPG	Ongoing	500+	Yes	Yes	?
Lejeune et al	1989	182 (Stage I and II) ? Nos	No	No	92% + 53.5% 5 year survival

At St Mary's Hospital, London, between 1980 and 1990, 42 patients with poor risk malignant melanoma of the extremities were subjected to isolated limb perfusion. Of these patients six had melanomas of the upper limb and 36 in the lower limb. From the time of inception of the MRC trial (taken over after two years by the British Association of Surgical Oncology and then the Melanoma Study Group) these patients were entered but sadly due to poor accrual, the trial was closed in 1988. All these patients had a malignant melanoma greater than 1.7 mm in thickness situated on a lower limb. There was no mortality and the morbidity was extremely low.

Fortunately, the WHO Melanoma Programme and the EORTC organized a prospective randomized clinical trial for all patients with Stage I malignant

melanoma on a limb with a Breslow thickness greater than 1.5 mm. The design of
the clinical trial is shown in Table 10.3. Originally, this study was to have closed
after the accrual of 500 patients. It has now been extended and therefore the
results are not yet available. In 1986, the North American Perfusion Group
(NAPG) collaborated with this trial. To date, no major complication has been
described in the perfusion group.

Table 10.3. Design of clinical trial

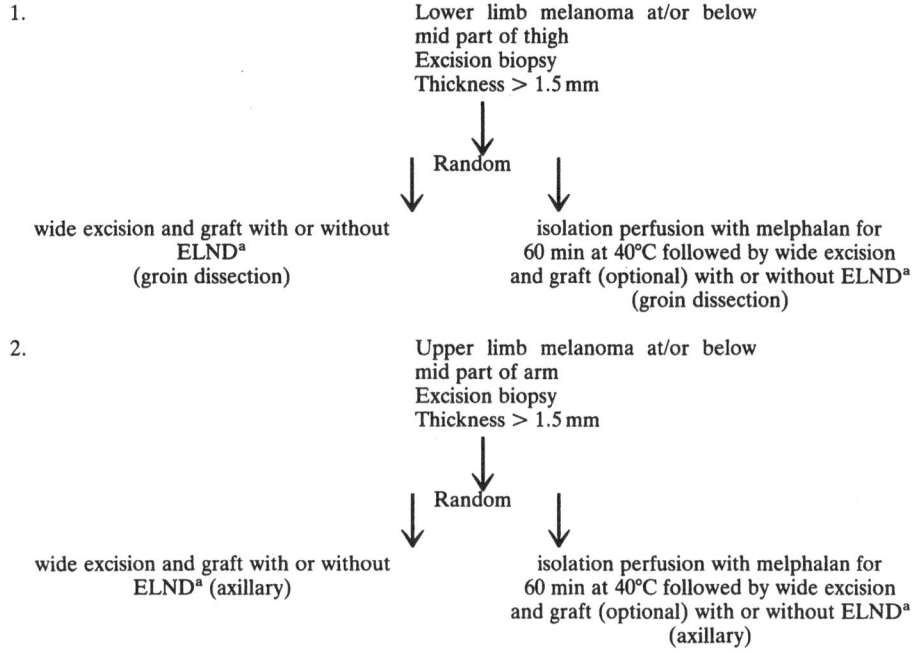

| 1. | Lower limb melanoma at/or below mid part of thigh
Excision biopsy
Thickness > 1.5 mm |

Random

wide excision and graft with or without ELND[a] (groin dissection)

isolation perfusion with melphalan for 60 min at 40°C followed by wide excision and graft (optional) with or without ELND[a] (groin dissection)

| 2. | Upper limb melanoma at/or below mid part of arm
Excision biopsy
Thickness > 1.5 mm |

Random

wide excision and graft with or without ELND[a] (axillary)

isolation perfusion with melphalan for 60 min at 40°C followed by wide excision and graft (optional) with or without ELND[a] (axillary)

[a] ELND (elective lymph node dissection) is optional but the same policy must be followed by the
participating centres through the whole trial. Stratifications will be made by centre. In case of ELND,
if lymph node micrometastases are discovered, the patient must be treated according to the protocol
and not excluded.

Conclusions

Isolated limb perfusion has been widely used in many hospitals worldwide over
the last 30 years. The rationale for isolated perfusion, as developed by Creech et
al. (1959), was to increase the chemotherapeutic dose in the isolated area beyond
that which could be obtained systemically and to avoid systemic toxicity. The
concentration of drugs could be safely increased from 6 to 10 times that given
systemically. This has been well and truly proven. Elevating the Po_2 tension has
been found to potentiate the effect of alkylating agents on tumour cells as has the
addition of hyperthermia which also raises the metabolic rate and produces better
perfusion by dilatation.

Indications for perfusion are as an adjunct to primary surgical treatment and also for the treatment of recurrent disease. The efficacy of isolated limb perfusion in the former group, i.e. prophylactic isolated limb perfusion, has been reported by many different centres but is yet to be proved by prospective randomized trial. The WHO-EORTC-NAPG trial should give an answer in the near future. There is less controversy for the treatment of patients with recurrent melanoma. Isolated perfusion is well accepted as the treatment of choice for recurrent malignant melanoma of the limbs.

References

Aigner K, Hild P, Henneking K, Paul E, Hundeiker M (1983) Regional perfusion with cis-platinum and dacarbazine. Recent Results Cancer Res 86:239–245

Au F, Goldman L (1977) Isolation perfusion in limb melanoma: a critical assessment and literature review. In: Clark WH, Goldman LI, Mastrangelo MJ (eds.) Human malignant melanoma. Grune and Stratton, New York, pp 295–308

Cavaliere R, Ciocatto E, Giovanella B et al. (1967) Selective heat sensitivity of cancer cells: biochemical and clinical studies. Cancer 20:1351–1381

Cavaliere R, Calabra A, Di Fillippo F, Carlini S, Giovannella B (1987) Prognostic parameters in limb recurrent melanoma treated with hypothermic antiblastic perfusion (Abstract). ICRCT, Ulm, G7:167

Creech O, Ryan R, Krementz ET (1959) Treatment of malignant melanoma by isolation perfusion technique. JAMA 169:339–343

Davis CD, Ivans JC, Soule EH (1975) Mayo Clinic experience with isolated perfusion for invasive malignant melanoma of the extremities. Proceedings of the Ninth International Pigment Cell Conference, Houston. S Karger, New York, p 379

Franklin H, Schraffordt Koops H, Oldhoff H et al. (1988) To perfuse or not to perfuse? A retrospective comparative study to evaluate the effect of adjuvant isolated regional perfusion in patients with stage I extremity melanoma with a thickness of 1.5 mm or greater. J Clin Oncol 6:705–708

Ghussen F, Negle K, Groth W, Müller JM, Stützer H (1984) A prospective randomized study of regional extremity perfusion in patients with malignant melanoma. Ann Surg 200:764–768

Ghussen F, Kruger I, Groth W, Stützer H (1988) The role of regional hyperthermic cystostatic perfusion in the treatment of extremity melanoma. Cancer 61:654–659

Golomb FM (1976) Perfusion of melanoma: 133 isolated perfusions in 114 patients. Panminerva Med 18:8–10

Hartley JW, Fletcher WS (1987) Improved survival of patients with stage II melanoma of the extremities using hyperthermic isolation perfusion with L-phenylalanine mustard. J Surg Oncol 36:170–174

Hoekstra HJ, Baas PC, Schraffordt Koops H, Oldhoff J (1989) Improved results of hypothermic isolation perfusion (hip) of locally metstasised melanoma of the lower extremities with melphalan with or without dactinomycin using different methods and dosage. Proc Ann Meet Am Soc Clin Oncol 8:A1093

Illig L, Aigner K (1980) Therapie des malignen Malanoms unter besonderer Berucksichtigung der isolierten Extremitatenperfusion. Dt Arztebl 77:2911–2925

Israels SP (1987) Loco-regional drug delivery in cancer treatment, with special reference to isolation perfusion. In: Veronesi U (ed.) Drug delivery in cancer treatment. Springer, Berlin, pp 53–76

Jonsson P, Hafstrom L, Hugander A (1983) Results of regional perfusion for primary and recurrent melanomas of the extremities. Recent Results Cancer Res 86:277–282

Klopp C, Alford T, Bateman J, Berry G, Winship T (1950) Fractionated intra-arterial cancer chemotherapy with bis-amine hydrochloride: a preliminary report. Ann Surg 132:811–832

Krementz ET (1986) Lucy Wortham James lecture. Regional perfusion. Current sophistication, what next. Cancer 57:416–432

Krementz ET (1987) Regional perfusion for melanoma of the limbs: prospects for cooperative studies in North America. In: Veronesi U, Cascinelli N, Santinami M (eds.) Cutaneous melanoma; status of knowledge and future perspectives. Academic Press, London, pp 589–602

Krementz ET, Ryan RF, Carter RD, Sutherland CM, Reed RJ (1985) Hyperthermic regional perfusion for melanoma of the limbs. In: Balch CM, Milton G (eds.) Cutaneous melanoma. Lippincott, Philadelphia, pp 172–195

Kroon BBR (1988) Regional isolation perfusion in melanoma of the limbs: accomplishments, unsolved problems, future. Eur J Surg Oncol 14:101–110

Lejeune FJ (1987) Is isolation perfusion with chemotherapy an improvement in the management of malignant melanoma? In: Kroon BBR, van Dongen JA (eds.) Oncologisch kabinet. A van Leeuwenhoek Huis, Nederlands Kanker Institut, Amsterdam, pp 71–78

Lejeune FJ, Ghanem GE (1987) A simple and accurate new method for cytostatic dosimetry in isolation perfusion of the limbs based on exchangeable blood volume determination. Cancer Res 47:639–643

Lejeune FJ, Deloof T, Ewalenko P et al. (1983) Objective regression of unexcised melanoma in-transit metastases after hyperthermic isolation perfusion of the limbs with melphalan. Recent Results Cancer Res 86:268–276

Lejeune FJ, Lienard D, Douaihy M, Vadoud Seyedi J, Ewalenko P (1989) Results of 206 isolated limb perfusions for malignant melanoma. Eur J Surg Oncol 15:510–519

Luck J (1956) Action of p-di(2-chloroethyl)-amino-L-phenylalanine on Harding Passey mouse melanoma. Science 123:984–985

Martijn H, Oldhoff J, Schraffordt Koops H (1981) Regional perfusion in the treatment of patients with a locally metastasized malignant melanoma of the limbs. Eur J Cancer 70:471–476

Martijn H, Oldhoff J, Schraffordt Koops H, Oosterhuis JW (1982) Hyperthermic regional perfusion with melphalan and a combination of melphalan and actinomycin-D in the treatment of locally metastasized malignant melanoma of the extremities. J Surg Oncol 20:9–13

Martijn H, Schraffordt Koops H, Milton GW et al. (1986) Comparison of two methods of treating primary malignant melanomas Clark IV and V, thickness 1.5 mm and greater, localized on the extremities. Cancer 57:1923–1930

McBride CM, Sugarbaker EV, Hickey RC (1975) Prophylactic isolation–perfusion as the primary therapy for invasive malignant melanoma of limbs. Ann Surg 182:316–324

McBride C, Smith L, Brown B (1981) Primary malignant melanoma of the limbs: a re-evaluation using microstaging techniques. Cancer 48:1463–1468

Rege VB, Leone LA, Soderberg CH jun. et al. (1983) Hyperthermic adjuvant perfusion chemotherapy for Stage I malignant melanoma of extremities, with literature review. Cancer 52:2033–2039

Rochlin D, Smart C (1965) Treatment of malignant melanoma by regional perfusion. Cancer 18:1544–1550

Rosin RD (1991) Treatment of cutaneous malignant melanoma. In: Taylor I, Johnson CD (Eds.) Recent advances in surgery, 14, Churchill Livingstone, Edinburgh pp 127–128

Rosin RD, Westbury C (1980) Isolated limb perfusion for malignant melanoma. Practitioner 224:188–198

Ryan RF, Krementz ET, Creech O, Winblad JW, Chamblee W, Cheek H (1957) Selected perfusion of isolated viscera with chemotherapeutic agents using extracorporeal circuit. Surg Forum 8:158–161

Schraffordt Koops H, Pldhoff J, Ploeg E van der, Vermey A, Eibergen R, Beekhuis H (1977) Some aspects of the treatment of primary malignant melanoma of the extremities by isolated regional perfusion. Cancer 39:27–33

Schraffordt Koops H, Beekhuis H, Oldhoff J, Oosterhuis J, Ploeg E van der, Vermey A (1981). Local recurrence and survival in patients with (Clark's level IV/V and over 1.5 mm thickness) stage I malignant melanoma of the extremities after regional perfusion. Cancer 48:1952–1957

Schraffordt Koops H, Kroon BBR, Lejeune FJ (1990) Isolated regional perfusion in the treatment of local recurrence, satellites and in-transit metastases of extremity melanomas. In: Rumke P (ed.) Therapy of advanced malignant melanoma, vol 10. Pigment cell series. Karger, Basel

Shiu MH, Knapper WH, Fortner JG et al. (1986) Regional isolated limb perfusion of melanoma intransit metastases using mechlorethamine (nitrogen mustard). J Clin Oncol 4:1819–1826

Stehlin J, Clark R, White EC et al. (1960) Regional chemotherapy for cancer: experiences with 116 perfusions. Ann Surg 151:605–619

Stehlin JS jun. (1980) Hyperthermic perfusion for melanoma of the extremities: experience with 165 patients, 1967–1979. Ann NY Acad Sci 335:352–355

Stehlin JS, Greef PJ, de Ipolyi PD (1988) Heat as an adjuvant in the treatment of advanced melanoma: an immune stimulant? Houston Med J 4:61–82

Storm FK, Morton DL (1985) Value of therapeutic hyperthermic limb perfusion in advanced recurrent melanoma of the lower extremity. Am J Surg 150:32–35

Sugarbaker EV, McBride CM (1976) Survival and regional disease control after isolation–perfusion for invasive Stage I melanoma of extremities. Cancer 37:181–198

Tonak J, Hohenberger W, Weidner F, Gohl H (1983) Hyperthermic perfusion in malignant melanoma: 5-year results. Recent Results Cancer Res 86:229–238

Vaglini M, Ammatuna M, Nava M et al. (1983) Regional perfusion at high temperature in the treatment of stage IIIA–IIIAB melanoma patients. Tumori 69:585–588

Vaglini M, Belli F, Marolda R, Prada A, Santinami M, Cascinelli N (1987) Hyperthermic antiblastic perfusion with DTIC in stage III–IIIAB melanoma of the extremities. Eur J Surg Oncol 13:127–129

Wieberdink J, Benckhuizen C, Braat RP, Slooten EA van, Olthuis GA (1982) Dosimetry in isolation perfusion of the limbs by assessment of perfused tissue volume and grading of toxic reactions. Eur J Cancer Clin Oncol 18:905–910

11 Systemic Treatment of Metastatic Malignant Melanoma

E. Sheridan and B. W. Hancock

Introduction

Surgery may be curative in low risk localized malignant melanoma. However, once a tumour has metastasized the outlook is inexorably bad. Almost all patients will eventually die and the median survival is still in terms of months! Against this gloomy scenario there has been a relentless search for systemic therapies which could prove effective in metastatic disease. Improved survival is the ultimate aim, but meanwhile palliation remains of the essence in our care of patients.

Single Agent Regimes

Dacarbazine (DTIC)

Dacarbazine has long been acknowledged to be the gold standard against which new systemic therapies for metastatic malignant melanoma should be measured.

In 1972 Wagner et al. reported on 393 patients treated with intravenous (i.v.) DTIC in a dose of 4.5 mg/kg/day for 10 days. The overall response rate in the trial was 28%. This response rate has never been bettered in any large-scale trial of single agent therapy, and indeed all later trials reported lower response rates such that an aggregate 21% has been quoted for DTIC regimes generally (Balch et al. 1989). Responses are on the whole of short duration with a median time to relapse of 5–6 months. Single agent DTIC is well tolerated, the dose-limiting toxicity is myleosuppression, but in standard regimes no more than 5% of patients are reported to have white cell nadirs of $<1.0 \times 10^9$/l or platelet nadirs of $<20 \times 10^9$/l. All patients have transient elevations of liver transaminases and rarely a life-threatening hepatic failure occurs. Nausea and vomiting are very common but well controlled by single agent antiemetic regimes.

The usually recommended regimes are:
1. 850 mg/m^2 i.v.   3 weekly
2. 250 mg/m^2/day   i.v. $\times$ 5   3 weekly
3. 4.5 mg/m^2/day   i.v. $\times$ 10   4 weekly

Nitrosureas

This group of agents also has a defined action against melanoma; the aggregate response is around 10%–18% (Balch et al. 1989). The most studied of the group are lomustine (CCNU) and carmustine (BCNU) often in combination regimes, and a new member of this class, fotemustine, has recently become available and has shown valuable activity in the treatment of disseminated melanoma.

Despite the lipid solubility of the nitrosoureas and their ability to cross the blood–brain barrier, the older agents did not show any activity against cerebral disease, however, there are now well validated reports of the effectiveness of fotemustine in this respect (Jacquillat et al. 1990a, b).

Fotemustine is a new nitrosourea which covalently deactivates the thioredoxin glutathione and ribonucleotide reductases. It is thought that the inhibition of these electron transfer systems is the basis for the cytotoxicity of the agent (Schallreuter et al. 1990). It has been shown that thioredoxin reductase (TR) is preferentially inactivated and it has been proposed that tumours with high TR levels would be most sensitive to the agent (Schallreuter and Wood, 1991).

A total of 153 patients have been evaluated in a French multicentre trial of 169 patients (Jacquillat et al. 1990a) of which 40% had had no prior chemotherapy; all had a Karnofsky of >60%. As fotemustine may cross the blood–brain barrier, patients with cerebral disease were eligible for the study and constituted 23.5% of entrants.

Patients received 100 mg/m^2 i.v. weekly for three weeks followed 4–5 weeks later by 100 mg/m^2 i.v. every three weeks until progression. There were three complete responses (CRs, complete resolution of clinical and investigational abnormalities) and 34 partial responses (PRs, > 50% improvement) – an overall 24.2% response rate with median duration of response of 22 weeks. Nine patients responded at cerebral sites and there were also responses in visceral (including lung) and non-visceral sites. Previously untreated patients responded better than previously treated patients, and less response was seen in those previously treated with other nitrosoureas.

Toxicity was principally haematological with leucopenia seen in 46.3% and thrombocytopenia in 40.3% of patients. Some nausea and vomiting were experienced by all patients as were transient elevations of liver eynzymes.

Vindesine

Promising phase one trials prompted the use of vindesine as a single agent in advanced melanoma. The South-Western Oncology Group (SWOG) (Quagliana et al. 1984) reported on 42 patients (24 female, 18 male) treated at a dose of 3 mg/m^2 by slow i.v. push at 7–14-day intervals, doses being adusted to give the maximum tolerated dose as frequently as possible. Of 34 evaluable patients there was 1 CR and 7 PRs, an overall response rate of 20%. Four responders were male, four were female; there were no responses outside of lymph node, subcutaneous or pulmonary sites. Responses were of 2–12 months duration.

Retsas et al. (1985) reported on a group of 65 patients, 57 of whom had Stage III disease, treated at the same dose of vindesine weekly for six weeks. Although this group of patients is not strictly comparable with those treated by the SWOG as there were patients with Stage III disease in the study group, the overall response rate was again 20%.

Toxicity with this regime is principally haematological and neurological. In the SWOG trial there were leucocyte nadirs of $<2.0 \times 10^9/l$ in nine and moderate or severe peripheral neuropathy in eight patients.

Detrorubicin

An anthracycline which differs from doxorubicin only in the C-14 side chain, detrorubicin has a strikingly different pharmacology, and unlike doxorubicin has been reported to have significant activity in melanoma, although experience with its use is still sparse. .

Chawla et al. (1985) reported on 42 patients each of whom received a 30 min i.v. infusion in doses of 120–180 mg/m² every three weeks. Although there were no CRs in the trial there were seven PRs, an overall rate of 19%. The principal sites of response were soft tissue and lymph node.

Surprisingly perhaps, in view of the other marked differences between detrorubicin and doxorubicin, it shares the latter's toxicities. Mild to moderate nausea and vomiting were experienced by 43% of patients, leucopenia by 78% and thrombocytopenia by 15%. Three patients experienced falls in left ventricular ejection fraction of greater than 50%, at cumulative doses of 1040–1620 mg/m². Only one of these patients, who received a total dose of 1290 mg/m², developed clinical cardiac failure; this responded well to digoxin and diuretics.

Taxol

Taxol is derived from the bark of the Pacific yew; it is the first agent with a taxene ring demonstrated to have antineoplastic properties. It binds preferentially to polymerized intracellular tubulin and stabilizes it, inhibiting the normal dynamic reorganization of the microtubule network. This results in the formation of bundles of disorganized microtubules and excessive numbers of abnormal asters during mitosis. Transition from the G to S phase is then prevented; taxol is also reported to have inhibitory effects during interphase itself (Rowinsky et al. 1990). Antineoplastic activity has been reported in refractory ovarian cancer; the Gynaecologic Oncology Group reports an overall 37% response rate (Thigpen et al. 1990).

Wiernik et al. (1987) treated 34 patients with advanced melanoma with a continuous infusion of taxol 250 mg/m² three weekly. There were two CRs and three PRs, an overall 15% response rate. Legha et al. (1990b) treated 25 patients with the same regime; there were no CRs and only three PRs (12% overall response). Three further patients experienced measurable regression short of PR or had stabilization of disease. In those in whom an objective regression was seen, progression did not occur until 6–17 months later. This durability was not a feature of the report by Wiernik et al. (1987), although one of their CRs was maintained for 14 months. All other responses were of short duration.

Both groups found toxicity to be mild at these doses. Myelosuppression is the major dose-limiting effect, neutropenic nadir occurring by day 8–11. Recovery is usually rapid and hospital admission due to fever is uncommon. The neutropenia does not appear cumulative and was experienced by 64% and 68% of Legha and Wiernik's patients respectively. A peripheral sensory neuropathy was experienced by 59% and 64% of patients. This usually takes the form of a glove and stocking numbness; it does appear cumulative but usually resolves within months of discontinuation of treatment. In both these studies severe bone pain was experienced by all patients, starting 2–3 days after treatment; several patients required narcotic analgesia.

Phase 2 studies had reported fatal anaphylaxis; however, administration as a continuous infusion and pretreatment with dexamethasone and diphenylhydramine appears to obviate the problem (Rowinsky et al. 1990).

Dibromodulcitol

A cytotoxic brominated hexitol, dibromodulcitol has found use in a variety of advanced malignancies. It is thought to act by inhibition of chromatin proteins and proteoglycan biosynthesis. It has been used as a single agent and in combinations in melanoma.

Bellet et al. (1978) treated 25 patients at a dose of $100 \, mg/m^2/day \times 10$ and the same regimen was used in a further 25 patients by Simmonds et al. (1985). In all there were two CRs and nine PRs, an overall response rate of 22%; responses were seen at visceral and soft tissue sites and were seen (in the report by Bellet's group) in patients previously treated with DTIC and nitrosoureas.

In contrast Medina and Kirkwood (1982) and Murray et al. (1985) have treated 41 patients and seen no responses. The reasons for this discrepancy are unclear, although seven of Medina and Kirkwood's patients had brain metastases and the cumulative dose given was lower than in the first two studies and Murray's study was of patients all previously treated; both groups saw rapid progression of disease while on treatment.

The latest reports of dibromodulcitol in combination with DTIC as a maintenance regime have quoted a 17% response rate (Gentile et al. 1988).

The principal toxicity of this agent is myelosuppression, reported to be significant at cumulative dose levels of $1500–1800 \, mg/m^2$ and more common with daily than intermittent regimes.

Summary

Few of the later reports have demonstrated response rates as good as those originally reported by Wagner et al. (1972).

Detrorubicin has an aggregate of 19% responses which compares well with 21% with DTIC; however, the initial reports of 22% response rate for dibromodulcitol have not been borne out by later studies. The risk of cardiac toxicity with detrorubicin is not trivial and its profile is not otherwise sufficiently advantageous to presently recommend it over DTIC.

In contrast fotemustine appears to offer a treatment option in those patients with cerebral disease, a site where hitherto there have been few reports of response. The French multicentre trial (Jacquillat et al. 1990 a, b) of reasonably large numbers is now backed up by other reports of good response to this agent (Aamdal et al. 1990) and it must therefore be regarded as a very useful addition to the armamentarium.

Features favouring a response were recognized early on. Costanza et al. (1977) stated that in their trial of DTIC and nitrosoureas favourable characteristics were female sex, young age, absence of CNS and visceral metastases and no prior chemotherapy. These features also hold for the later agents; all eight responses to detrorubicin, the majority of those to taxol and most of those to dibromodulcitol have been in previously untreated patients.

Alone of the more recent agents fotemustine seems to provide a hope of response in those with brain disease, and also appears to overcome visceral resistance to treatment in a proportion of patients.

Combination Regimes

As late as 1985 it was the general opinion that combination regimes had failed to demonstrate any advantage compared to DTIC alone (Balch et al. 1989). In general toxicity was greater and there was no obvious benefit in terms of response or survival (Lakhani et al. 1990).

In this chapter regimes with a reported response rate in excess of 40% are reviewed; results are, however, not consistent with any one regime in different hands and several of the combinations have been evaluated by different groups with strikingly different results.

DTIC/Lomustine/Cisplatin/Tamoxifen

Del Prete et al. (1984) treated 20 patients with cisplatin $25 \, mg/m^2/day$ and DTIC $220 \, mg/m^2/day$ for three days every 3 weeks, lomustine $150 \, mg/m^2$ every six weeks and tamoxifen 10 mg bd daily. There were four CRs and seven PRs in the group, a 55% overall response rate. One of these died at 7 months of lomustine toxicity, but the others all achieved responses of more than 14 months duration. Duration of PR was 3–15 months. All four CRs occurred in lung disease (one also had bone disease). There were only five men in the trial and eight of the responses were in women.

McClay and colleagues (McClay and Mastrangelo 1988; McClay et al. 1987, 1989) have treated a total of 42 patients with the regime; 39 were evaluable and there have been four CRs and 15 PRs for an overall response rate of 49%. Many of the responses appear durable; two of the original CRs were still in remission 3.5 years later (McClay and Mastrangelo, 1988). Interestingly in their original group of 23 patients, only four of the 10 responders were female whereas the original del Prete group had predominantly female entry and responders. Only one of these 10 responders had previously been treated with chemotherapy.

Toxicity in this latter trial was mild: 55% of patients had a leucopenia of less than $3.0 \times 10^9/l$ and 30% less than $1.0 \times 10^9/l$; 35% had platelets less than $50 \times 10^9/l$; one patient with a platelet count of $6 \times 10^9/l$ required platelet transfusion. Reversible elevations in serum creatinine were also seen but it was the myelosuppression which was dose limiting and resulted in most patients receiving 4-weekly rather than 3-weekly DTIC/cisplatin.

In the original study six of 20 patients developed deep vein thromboses (DVTs) and there were two pulmonary emboli (PEs). Five of the six were responders. Tamoxifen reduces antithrombin III levels and was eliminated from a subsequent study of 20 patients by the group. There were no DVTs or PEs in this study but the response rate was only 10%. Thus although tamoxifen has little activity on its own in melanoma it appears to be an important component of the regime.

It is felt by these authors that the calcium channel blocking action of tamoxifen is the basis for its synergism with cisplatin, as in animal models the combination of cisplatin and verapamil results in tumour regression at lower does of cisplatin than when the agent is used on its own (Oneda et al. 1990). It is known that melanoma cells have a high aromatase activity (Santen et al. 1988) and that oestrogen biosynthesis is possible, and it has also been shown that inhibition of such activity does not improve the efficacy of DTIC alone (Harvey et al. 1988). However, melanoma cells do express the oestrogen receptor protein in about 50% of patients (Walker et al. 1987), thus although inhibition of local oestrogen action may not be of any significance to the action of tamoxifen this does not preclude some, as yet unidentified, clinically significant effect as a consequence of its interaction with the oestrogen receptor.

Bleomycin/Oncovin/Lomustine/DTIC (BOLD)

A total of 91 consecutive patients with Stage IV melanoma, some of whom had received prior chemotherapy were treated with bleomycin 7.5 units subcutaneously (s.c.) days 1 and 4, vincristine 1 mg/m^2 i.v. days 1 and 5, lomustine 80 mg/m^2 orally on day 1 and DTIC 200 mg/m^2 i.v. days 1–5 (Seigler et al. 1980).

A total of 72 patients were available for evaluation and there were seven CRs and 22 PRs – an overall 40% response rate. The median duration of response was 30 weeks with median survival of 87 weeks in responders and 20 weeks in non-responders.

These results could not be reproduced by a further trial of 51 patients treated with the same regime by the Prudente Foundation (1989). Some of these had had prior chemotherapy but there were only two PRs, both short lived, and the median duration of survival for all patients who received at least two cycles of treatment (an evaluation criterion in Seigler's study) was 17.3 weeks with an approximate 95% confidence limit of 23 weeks – much lower than the overall 30-week survival for the original BOLD report. From the data published neither study appears unbalanced for any known prognostic factor. Although 82% of the Prudente group had visceral disease it is not stated whether this was predominantly outside the lungs. The only other factor likely to be of significance is that 42 patients presented with disseminated disease, and no prior surgery, in this group.

The results of the Royal Marsden group with the BOLD protocol have recently been republished by Lakhani et al. (1990) who achieved an overall 24.4% response rate similar to that reported by York and Foltz (1988).

The dose-limiting toxicity in the report by Seigler et al. (1980) was myelo-suppression; it was moderate (leucocytes $<1.0 \times 10^9$/l and platelets $<100 \times 10^9$/l) in 36% of patients. Nausea and vomiting were moderate or severe in 40%.

Bleomycin/Eldesine/Lomustine/DTIC (BELD)

The very similar BELD regime has been assessed by Young et al. (1985) in 21 patients with Stage III melanoma. All but three patients had had no prior chemotherapy. Vindesine was substituted for vincristine because of the very poor response rate reported with the latter as a single agent. All patients had two or more cycles of bleomycin 15 mg s.c. days 1 and 4, vindesine 3 mg/m^2 i.v. days 1 and 5, lomustine 80 mg/m^2 orally day 1 (max. 150 mg) and DTIC 200 mg/m^2 (max. 400 mg) i.v. days 1–5. There were three CRs (all females with pulmonary or subcutaneous disease) and six PRs (four male, two female) – 45% overall response. The CRs were of 12, 16 and 52 weeks ongoing duration, the PRs of 8–52 weeks duration, and the median survival in responders was 43 weeks compared with a median survival of 15 weeks in non-responders. All but two responses were in pulmonary or subcutaneous tissue.

Toxicity was moderate; most patients experienced nausea and vomiting and significant alopecia occurred in more than 50%. Only four of 21 experienced significant myelosuppression although all had transient leucopenia (leucocytes $<2.5 \times 10^9$/l).

Cisplatin/Vindesine/Dacarbazine

Gundoroon (1987) evaluated 27 patients treated with cisplatin 100 mg/m^2 and vindesine 3 mg/m^2 both i.v. on day 1, DTIC 250 mg/m^2 i.v. days 1–5; 13 patients had received prior chemotherapy. There were four CRs and eight PRs (44% overall); seven of 17 males responded and five of 10 females. All four CRs were in lung, and the majority of PRs were in lung or soft tissue. A further 27 patients were treated with a similar regime by Pectasides et al. (1989); none had had prior chemotherapy. There were four CRs and eight PRs (45% overall) and all responses were in lung or soft tissue. There were no hepatic responses and no data were given on the sex of responders. Duration of CR was 2–10 months and of PR 3–18 months in these two studies

Verschraegen et al. (1988) used DTIC 450 mg/m^2, vindesine 3 mg/m^2 and cisplatin 50 mg/m^2 all i.v. on days 1 and 8, courses repeated 4 weekly. A total of 105 patients were treated with 92 being evaluable. There were four CRs and 18 PRs (24% overall response rate) with median duration of 23 weeks. Of 46 men nine responded compared with 13 of 24 women; three of 22 responders had received prior chemotherapy compared with 22 of 70 non-responders and 75% of responses were in skin, lymph nodes or lungs. Of particular note in this study was the 32% incidence of liver metastases at entry and the development of symptoma-tic brain metastases by 33 patients whilst on trial. No stabilization of these metastases ever occurred and in 15, progression occurred even in the presence of peripheral tumour response.

Evaluation was very full in this study and the relatively low response rate may be explained by the high incidence of resistant liver disease at entry and the subsequent high incidence of brain metastases.

Toxicity with the regime is not inconsiderable: Verschraegen et al. (1988) report universal nausea, vomiting and diarrhoea: WHO grade 3 or 4 leucopenia was seen in 23 patients, alopecia occurred in 56% of patients, peripheral neuropathy in 33% and nephrotoxicity in 17%.

A similar regime of vinblastine 1.6 mg/m² day i.v. for 5 days, DTIC 800 mg/m² i.v. on day 1 and cisplatin 20 mg/m²/day i.v. on days 2–6, at 3-weekly intervals was studied by Legha et al. (1989) in 52 patients. There were two CRs and 18 PRs in 50 evaluable patients, an overall response rate of 40%. Seventeen patients had objective regression at hepatic sites though not all were PR or CR. Median duration of response was 9 months and the median survival of responders was 12 months compared with 6 months in non-responders. There was no regression of brain metastases but five patients did achieve temporary stabilization. Toxicity was similar to that seen with the vindesine stabilization. Toxicity was similar to that seen with the vindesine combination.

An earlier EORTC study of vindesine/DTIC versus DTIC alone achieved an overall response rate of 25% for the combination and 18% for vindesine alone (Mulder et al. 1982). The EORTC group felt the addition of cisplatin to the regimen had not improved response but significantly increased toxicity (Verschraegen et al. 1988).

Procarbazine/Oncovin/Carmustine (POC)

Carmo-Pereira et al. (1984) reported on 44 patients (nine previously untreated) treated with procarbazine 100 mg/m² p.o. (max. 150 mg) days 1–10, vincristine 1.4 mg/m² i.v. (max. 2 mg) days 1 and 8 and carmustine 150 mg/m² p.o. (max. 200 mg) on day 1 at 4–6 week intervals. There were 11 CRs and 10 PRs; 13 of 24 males and 8 of 20 females responded. Responses were only seen in skin, lymph nodes or lung.

Following this Shelley et al. (1985) treated 65 previously untreated patients with the same regime but there were only seven responders overall. This was a well-conducted study with a 50:50 male/female ratio in young (median age 52 years) patients. Performance status was not an exclusion criterion in this study, as it was (Karnofsky > 50%; patient ambulatory and at least fit enough not to require major assistance in daily living and self-care) in the Carmo-Pereira study. The results were obviously disappointing but the authors felt that this could be explained by the preponderance of visceral disease in their group (83% of patients) compared with 36% in the earlier study where 16 of 21 responses occurred in the 28 patients with no visceral disease. Of the eight responses in the Shelley study four were in the 11 patients with no visceral disease.

Dose-limiting toxicity was myelosuppression with 11% and 15% of the patients in the studies by Carmo-Pereira and Shelley suffering leucocyte counts of <2.0 × 10⁹/l and platelet counts of <100 × 10⁹/l respectively.

A further study of the regime (Evans et al. 1990) in which 27 fit young patients were treated there were three CRs and five PRs, 30% overall. Again responses were principally in skin, lung and at nodal sites.

DTIC/Fotemustine

Among 70 patients with disseminated melanoma who were treated by Avril et al. (1990) there were 63 evaluable patients who received fotemustine $100\,mg/m^2$ i.v. on days 1 and 8, and DTIC $250\,mg/m^2$ i.v. on days 15–18 followed by a 4–5 week rest. Patients with no progression received fotemustine $100\,mg/m^2$ on day 1 and DTIC $250\,mg/m^2$ on days 2–5 every 3 weeks. There were nine CRs and 12 PRs (33.3% overall). Among 20 previously treated patients there were seven responders; 28.6% of responses were at cerebral sites.

Aamdal et al. (1990) treated 30 patients with DTIC $500\,mg/m^2$, 3 h before fotemustine $100\,mg/m^2$, every 4 weeks. There were six patients with cerebral disease in this study and 13 with visceral disease. There were four CRs and four PRs (27% overall) with responses recorded principally at visceral sites. Less than 20% of patients experienced grade III or IV myelosuppression. One patient died with rapidly progressively pulmonary fibrosis.

A further 15 patients have been treated by Gore et al. (1991) with DTIC $250\,mg/m^2$ and fotemustine $100\,mg/m^2$ 2h later on days 1 and 8. After 3–5 weeks of rest the combination was repeated four weekly. Of 12 evaluable patients there were three PRs including one patient with cerebral metastasis. There was a significant but asymptomatic drop in lung diffusion capacity in one patient.

Summary

The overall experience with combination regimes suggests that improved responses can be obtained. However, it remains the case that the group of favourable characteristics previously outlined for single agent regimes still holds for the combination regimes; in particular the resistance of liver and brain disease to chemotherapy remains a major problem.

The success of individual centres with their own regimes should encourage multicentre trials to define further the clinical efficacy of these regimes. However, some authors feel that the superiority of combination regimes over single agents has now been established and would recommend their general use (McClay and Mastrangelo 1988).

Dose Intensification

Regimes using high doses of conventional cytotoxics have been developed since the recognition of the dose–response relationship for cytoxocity, i.e. that a linear increase in dose results in a log increase in cell kill. The toxicities in such regimes are severe, and attempts have been made to overcome them, such as in the use of autologous bone marrow transplantation in regimes with a profound myelo-suppressive action.

There are several reports of the use of such regimes in melanoma, both with and without marrow support.

Regimes Without Marrow Support

Lomustine/Vincristine/Melphalan

Eighteen patients previously untreated with chemotherapy and most with visceral-dominant disease (brain 8, liver 9) were treated by Tchekmedyian et al. (1986) with high dose lomustine 750 mg/m^2 i.v. on days 1, 2 and 3; vincristine 2 mg i.v. was given on days 1 and 8. Of these 18 patients six, whose marrow had recovered by 56 days, received melphalan 20 mg/m^2 daily for 3 days and further vincristine on days 1 and 8. There were no CRs and only one PR in this study which was associated with extreme toxicity. Five patients died of treatment-related complications (sepsis 2, cytomegalovirus pneumonia 1, *Pneumocystic carinii* pneumonia 1, myocardial infarct 1). There are no plans to use this regime further.

Cisplatin

A total of 38 patients were treated (Mortimer et al. (1990) with a dose of 200 mg/m^2/cycle. There was an overall response rate of 22%. A divided dose schedule (100 mg/m^2, days 1 and 8) was less toxic than a daily schedule; however, the response rate of 22% is no better than the response rate with DTIC alone.

Glover et al. (1987, 1989) have reported on the use of high dose cisplatinum together with the aminothiol WR2721, which in animal models protects against the renal, haematological and nervous system toxicities of cisplatin. Fifty-one patients were treated with cisplatin 100–150 mg/m^2 i.v. preceded 30 min earlier by 740–910 mg/m^2 i.v. of WR2721; treatment cycles were repeated at 3–4 weekly intervals. There were 21 PRs and two CRs, a 45% overall response rate. The majority of responses were in skin, lung or at nodal sites, but there were also seven responses in liver. There was a dose–response relationship for cisplatin. The use of the WR2721 appeared to reduce the amount of toxicity due to the cisplatin; transient nephrotoxicity was seen in only 9% of courses, and myelosuppression with platelet counts of <50 × 10^9/l in less than 6% of courses. There was also a marked reduction in the incidence of neuropathy and hearing loss.

Further trials are being co-ordinated under the auspices of the Eastern Cooperative Oncology Group (ECOG) to assess further the role of this agent in melanoma.

Autologous Bone Marrow Support

Melphalan

A total of 34 patients with predominantly visceral disease were treated by Cornbleet et al. (1983) with melphalan 140–260 mg/m^2 i.v. 7 days after cyclophosphamide priming with $300 \, mg/m^2$ i.v. Marrow was harvested on the day of treatment and reinfused 8–24 h after the administration of melphalan. Four patients received a further course of melphalan at a dose of $140 \, mg/m^2$ given after a convalescent period of at least 6 weeks. There were two CRs and five PRs (19%). In this group of patients there were seven deaths within one month of starting treatment; all patients experienced WHO grade 4 (life-threatening) myelosuppression and required 4 weeks of intensive support.

Lomustine

The same group treated nine further patients with high-dose lomustine $800 \, mg/m^2$ with marrow reinfusion at 48 h; there were three PRs and one CR in the study. There was only one death within one month of starting treatment. Grade 4 myelosuppression was seen in 50% of patients and grade 3 in 38%; overall 2 weeks of hospital stay was required. None of the patients in these two studies had had prior chemotherapy though there was a preponderance of patients with evidence of some visceral disease (Lakhani et al. 1990).

Dacarbazine (DTIC)

Thatcher et al. (1989) treated 34 patients with three i.v. regimes containing high-dose DTIC. Patients were allocated to receive regimes A, B or C on the basis of age and fitness. Only four patients had received prior chemotherapy.

> Young patients received:
> Regime A: DTIC $4.3–10.5 \, g/m^2$ followed by:
> > melphalan $30–65 \, mg/m^2 \times 2$ at 8 and 16 h later
>
> Older patients received either regime B or later regime C
> Regime B: DTIC $2.7–4.0 \, g/m^2$ followed by:
> > melphalan $15–20 \, mg/m^2$ at 8 and 16 h later
>
> Regime C: DTIC $7.0 \ 8.0 \, g/m^2$ followed by:
> > ifosfamide $2.5–4.0 \, g/m^2$ at 8 and 16 h later

Marrow was harvested immediately before chemotherapy and reinfused 12 h after the end of treatment. Of 17 patients 13 responded to regime A (CR 4, PR 9) with a median duration of response of 18 weeks. Three of 11 responded to regime B (CR 1, PR 2) and two of 10 responded to regime C (both PR). Median survival in A was 28 weeks, B 23 weeks and C 23 weeks. Responses were mainly in non-visceral, nodal and cutaneous sites.

Toxicity was severe; there were four deaths within 2 weeks of starting treatment, hospital stays were in excess of 3 weeks with all three regimes and there were no statistically significant differences between the regimes for mean time to blood count fall or recovery. No significant hepatic toxicities were recorded.

Lomustine/Cyclophosphamide/Cisplatin and Melphalan

In a phase I trial 29 patients were treated with the combination by Peters et al. (1986). There were 13 patients with melanoma. The i.v. regime was:

Day 1   Marrow harvest
Day 3   Cyclophosphamide 1500–5625 mg/m^2 (total dose days 3 and 6)
Day 3   Lomustine 150–750 mg/m^2
Day 3   Cisplatin 75–180 mg/m^2
Day 6   Cyclophosphamide 1500–5623 mg/m^2 (total dose days 3 and 6)

Seven patients who received dose-limiting levels of the above also received melphalan 40–80 mg/m^2/day.

There was one CR and seven PRs in the melanoma patients. The one CR died on day 75 of cytomegalovirus pneumonia; the PRs had durations of 2–10 months.

All patients experienced grade 4 myelosuppression and there were episodes of venocclusive disease in the study as a whole. The addition of melphalan to the regime profoundly increased the incidence of renal toxicity.

Summary

Overall the use of high dose regimens has been disappointing. Toxicities are predictably severe; responses are of limited duration and fail to confer a survival advantage on those receiving such regimes. Due to the long hospital stays and toxicities, quality of life is not improved consistently by their use.

These regimes have failed to overcome the resistance of bone and liver disease known to exist to more conventional regimes; they cannot at present be recommended for use.

Biological Therapy

Interferon

Single Agent Interferon

Recombinant interferons (IFN) became available and were being utilized on a large scale in trials by 1981. Both interferon α-2a (Roferon) and interferon α-2b (Intron) have been used in melanoma; there are no significant differences in results between the two agents.

Creagan et al. (1984) treated 31 patients with interferon α-2a 50 × 10^6 units/m^2 i.m. three times weekly (t.i.w.) for three months and a further 30 patients with 12 × 10^6 units/m^2 t.i.w.

Of the 61 patients 36 were regarded as good risk (ECOG 0, normal activity, or 1, symptomatic but ambulatory, with no prior chemotherapy). There were 40 males and 21 females. Overall there were four CRs and nine PRs (21% response rate). Three of the CRs and five of the PRs were in the good risk group; however, there was no statistically significant difference in response rates between patients stratified as good or poor risk. Responders had a median survival of 11.3 months compared with 6 months overall. A further update of the trial reported that three of the CRs, including one originally with liver disease, were still in remission at 49, 55 and 60 months (Creagan et al. 1987).

In contrast to the above Legha et al. (1987) reported only two PRs in a group of 31 patients treated with 18×10^6 units i.m. t.i.w. for 70 days, and three PRs in a further group of 35 patients (31 evaluable) treated with a daily schedule starting with interferon α-2a 3×10^6 units/day increased to 36×10^6 units/day over 12 days and then maintained until 70 days. Responses were principally in soft tissue, nodes and lungs and of durations of 27–88+ weeks. Hersey et al. (1985) report the treatment of 20 patients at doses of 15–50×10^6 units/m^2 t.i.w.; two patients showed complete remission.

All three groups found the higher doses of interferon to be associated with limiting toxicities taking the form of fever, fatigue, anaemia, myalgias and weight loss, leading to falls in performance status.

Another daily regime was studied by Neefe et al. (1990) in 97 evaluable patients. Interferon α-2a was given s.c. daily for 10 days, then the dose was escalated in four steps from 3×10^6 to 36×10^6 units/day over ten days. There were six CRs and two PRs (8%), the median duration of CR was 11 months, and no responses were seen in visceral disease outside the lungs.

Using interferon α-2b Dorval et al. (1986) reported on 24 patients given 10×10^6 units s.c. t.i.w. until disease progression. The median duration of treatment was 9 weeks (range 5–52 weeks) and 22 patients were available for evaluation. There were two CRs and four PRs (27% overall); the duration of CRs was 20 and 6 weeks.

A total of 63 patients were treated by Mughal et al. (1988) with 10×10^6 units/m^2 s.c. t.i.w.; 51 patients were evaluable for response and there were four CRs and six PRs (20% overall). All responses in this study were in soft tissue, lymph node or lungs (five of the six responses in the Dorval et al. trial were also in these sites) and the majority of responders were female.

A further trial by Mickiewicz et al. (1990) reported three CRs and three PRs among 16 patients (37.5% overall) treated with interferon α-2b 5–10×10^6 units daily for eight weeks; this was one arm of a two-armed trial comparing interferon α-2b alone with DTIC/interferon α-2b in combination.

The predominant toxicities reported by all groups are a flu-like illness and weight loss. Fever, fatigue, anorexia and myalgia constitute the flu-like illness; 80% of patients suffer fevers of 38.0°C or above but these can usually be controlled by paracetamol 500 mg 4–6 hourly. Nausea and vomiting occur in up to one-third of patients on the thrice weekly regime and altered taste sensation is reported by some patients. Elevation of liver enzymes and falls in platelet and white counts are seen though these are not usually of clinical significance.

The daily regimes and high dose regimes result in toxicity of such a degree as to reduce performance status and as there does not appear to be a dose-response relationship their use is not routinely recommended.

Interferon/DTIC

Following the encouraging results with interferon alone the Queensland group reported on the use of interferon with DTIC in 1987 (McLeod et al. 1987) and updated their results in 1990 (McLeod et al. 1990). A total of 76 patients (46 male, 30 female) were treated with interferon α-2a in a dosage escalated from 3×10^6 to

9×10^6 units/day over 70 days and then t.i.w. for a total of 6 months, combined with DTIC escalated from 200 to 800 mg/m^2 in increments every 21 days. Overall there was a 26% response rate (CRs 9%, PRs 17%). Only five patients had had prior chemotherapy and there were only two responses at visceral sites. The median duration of response was 52 weeks (range 11–166+) and of survival in these responders was 83 weeks (15–166+), compared with a median survival of the whole group of 43 weeks.

A further 30 patients (21 male, 9 female) were entered in a high-dose study and received interferon α-2a 18 × 10^6 units; the DTIC dosage remained the same. The ECOG status of 23 patients was 0–2 (at least fit enough to be out of bed more than 50% of the time) and only three had had prior chemotherapy. There were 7% CRs and 17% PRs (23% overall) with median duration of response 33 weeks (range 18–112+) and the median survival of responders was 56 weeks (range 37–112+). Toxicity was greater with the higher dose and four patients withdrew as a consequence.

Bajetta et al. (1990) treated 79 patients with interferon α-2a 9 × 10^6 units i.m. daily for 70 days and t.i.w. thereafter, plus DTIC 800 mg/m^2 three weekly for 6 months or until progression. In 75 evaluable patients, all with Karnofsky >70% (self-caring but limited normal activity) and no prior chemotherapy or CNS disease, there were six CRs (8%) and 13 PRs (17%), 25% overall. There were only three responses at visceral sites and mean duration of response was 8.2 ± 4.2 months. There was one treatment-related death due to sepsis after myelosuppression and dosage reduction due to toxicity was required in 12 patients.

Kirkwood et al. (1990) reported on 74 patients entered into a three-arm study of DTIC versus interferon α-2b versus DTIC + interferon α-2b. The combination was DTIC 250 mg/m^2 daily i.v. for 5 days every 3 weeks and interferon α-2b 30 × 10^6 units daily for 5 days every week for 3 weeks, then at 10 × 10^6 units/m^2 s.c. t.i.w. The single-agent regime used these doses alone. There were responses in five of 24 patients on DTIC alone, one of 23 on interferon α-2b alone and four of 21 on the combination. There have been three other short reports of single agent versus combination, outlined in Table 11.1.

Overall results from these studies document 253 patients treated with combinations of interferon/DTIC, with an overall 29.7% response rate. Toxicities are

Table 11.1. Reports of single agent and combination interferon treatment

Investigator (number of patients)	Patients treated	Response	
		CR%	Overall % CR + PR
Mickiewicz et al. (1990) (53 non randomized)	IFN α-2b	18.7	37.5
	IFN α-2b/DTIC	10.8	29.7
Vorobiof et al. (1989) (40 randomized)	DTIC	5.3	16
	DTIC/IFN α-2b	22.2	39
Falkson et al. (1990) (54 randomized)	DTIC	–	17
	DTIC/IFN α-2b	–	38

overall similar to those experienced by patients receiving interferon alone; however, myelosuppression is a more serious problem and has been the cause of dosage delay and modification.

Interferon/Cisplatin

There is a report on the use of interferon and cisplatin in 25 patients. Margolin et al. (1990) used cisplatin $40 \, mg/m^2$ i.v. bolus on days 1 and 8 and interferon α-2a 3 $\times 10^6$ units/m^2 s.c. days 1–5 and 8–12 repeated three weekly. There was an overall 25% response rate in 24 evaluable patients.

Summary

Present results seem to indicate that the combination of DTIC/interferon produces more responses than interferon alone in the setting of disseminated melanoma. Toxicities are manageable. The most effective regime has yet to be determined; however, with the reported superiority of interferon given on a t.i.w. rather than daily basis (McLeod et al. 1990) it may be that a standard 5 day regime of i.v. DTIC together with interferon t.i.w. would produce the best response rate with the least toxicity.

Interleukin-2 (IL-2)

IL-2 Single Agent

A large body of evidence has accrued on the use of IL-2 with ex vivo activation of "killer" cells, in the management of melanoma (Rosenberg et al. 1987) and this has been recently updated (Skornick et al. 1990). However, the use of IL-2 alone has also been reported and evidence presented for its activity in lower dose continuous infusion (CI) (West et al. 1988).

Parkinson et al. (1990) reported on 47 patients treated with an IL-2 regime identical to that originally developed for use in the IL-2 lymphokine activated killer (LAK) cell studies of the NCI (Rosenberg et al. 1987). Patients received two five-day courses of IL-2 at doses of 10^5 units/kg as a 15 min infusion every 8 h daily, one week apart. Patients were evaluated at four and eight weeks after treatment and if there was evidence of antitumour response, were retreated at 12-weekly intervals to a maximum of three treatments.

There was one early treatment-related death and there were two CRs and eight PRs (22% overall). Of the ten responders eight were male and seven had an ECOG status of 0–1; most had received no prior chemotherapy. Responses were principally in skin, lung and at nodal sites; the median duration of response was eight months although there were four well-sustained (>12 months) responses.

This response rate is comparable to the response rate seen in the early NCI IL-2/LAK trials. Toxicity was also similar and, as with the IL-2/LAK studies, was cumulative. Hypotension requiring dopamine or neosynephrine was experienced by 72% of patients and there were three documented myocardial infarcts. Renal toxicity was considerable, 32% of patients developing creatinine levels of five times normal and 58% oliguria or anuria of 8 h duration. Seven patients required intravenous antibiotics for central venous catheter sepsis, which was the cause of the one treatment-related death.

The SWOG has reported on 46 patients treated in an out-patient setting with IL-2 10×10^6 Cetus units/m^2 as an i.v. bolus three times weekly later reduced to 6×10^6 Cetus units/m^2. There were four PRs only (10% overall) among 42 evaluable patients; median duration of response was 8.3 months (Whitehead et al. 1989).

In contrast Legha et al. (1990a) in a phase I–II trial treated patients with 96 h CI every six weeks. Of the 17 patients entered, the first three received 3×10^6 Cetus units/m^2/day, the rest 4×10^6 Cetus units/m^2/day. There was only one PR in this study.

Toxicities with these latter two low-dose regimes are not inconsiderable, 15% of patients in the infusion group experiencing grade 3 or 4 hepatic or renal toxicity; this was also common in the out-patient regime in which serious cardiac and neurological impairment was also seen.

IL-2/Cyclophosphamide

Mitchell et al. (1988) report on the use of IL-2 and cyclophosphamide. This agent was used with the aim of selectively depressing the suppressor T cell populations prior to IL-2 usage, thereby preferentially encouraging expansion of LAK cell population unimpeded by suppressor influences. A total of 27 patients were treated with cyclophosphamide 350 mg/m^2 i.v. bolus followed 3 days later by IL-2 3.6×10^6 units/m^2 i.v. bolus daily for five days. The regime was repeated at weekly intervals. The majority of patients (17) had no prior chemotherapy and there were 16 males and 11 females in the group. In 24 evaluable patients there were five PRs and one CR (25% overall); mean duration of responses was 5 months. All but two of the documented 12 sites of response were in lung, lymph node or soft tissue; the CR did include the complete regression of eight large liver metastases in a female patient.

Fatigue, fever and nausea and vomiting were experienced by all patients and four required i.v. fluids for significant hypotension but generally the regime was well tolerated. Immunological studies could not confirm that the use of cyclophosphamide had indeed had a significant effect on preferential LAK expansion.

IL-2/Dacarbazine (DTIC)

Flaherty et al. (1990) treated 32 patients with DTIC 1.0 g/m^2 24 h CI every 28 days on day 1 and IL-2 as a 30 min infusion on days 15–19 and 22–26 in doses of $2–5 \times 10^6$ Cetus units/m^2. Patients with objective evidence of response were treated until either a complete response or progression occurred. Twenty eight patients had no prior chemotherapy, there were 21 male and 11 female and all had ECOG status 0–2. There were six PRs and one CR (22% overall), the majority of which were in non-visceral sites. There were no responses in three patients with brain metastases and none in five patients with pancreatic or splenic masses. The median duration of response was 4.7 months (2.0–22+ months) and median survival of responders was 22+ months, compared with 5.9+ months in non-responders.

The regime was given on an out-patient basis and there were only two hospital admissions, one for i.v. fluids for hypotension and one for transfusion following an upper gastrointestinal bleed while suffering a WHO grade 4 thrombocytopenia.

Severe fatigue, hypotension, arthralgia, nausea, vomiting and anorexia were the chief causes of dosage alteration.

Papadopolous et al. (1989) treated 30 patient with DTIC 200 mg/m^2/24 h CI on days 1–5 and IL-2 24 × 10^6 international units i.v. by 30 min infusion on days 1–5 and 8–12 every 28 days. There were 20 males and 10 females, all with ECOG status 0–2. Patients with objective evidence of a response were treated until either a CR or progression occurred. There were four CRs and six PRs (33% overall) with a median duration of 16 weeks. The majority of responders (7 of 10) were female and responses occurred principally in non-visceral sites (18 of 21 documented organ responses). Of note is the fact that four of the 10 responders developed CNS metastases while in peripheral remission.

Most treatment was out-patient; there were three hospital admissions due to pulmonary oedema, hypotension and supraventricular tachycardia (one case each).

Stoter et al. (1989) treated 27 patients with an induction/maintenance regime. Patients received two induction cycles of IL-2 3 × 10^6 Cetus units/m^2/day as CI on days 1–15 and 12–17 with DTIC 850 mg/m^2 i.v. bolus on day 26, at 5-weekly intervals. Maintenance was 3 × 10^6 Cetus units/m^2/day for 5 days alternating with DTIC 850 mg/m^2 three weekly for 18 weeks. All had Karnofsky scores of 80%–100% (normal activity with effort, or normal) and only one had had prior chemotherapy. Of 24 evaluable patients there were four PRs and one CR (20.8% overall). This study did report a high proportion of responses in liver metastases. There were four treatment interruptions due to hypotension.

The toxicities experienced by patients on DTIC/IL-2 regimes are generally well tolerated; hypotension is the commonest cause of active intervention although treatment interruptions due to fatigue, arthralgia and anorexia are not uncommon. Significant granulocytopenia has been reported in 10% of patients but recovery from nadir counts is seen despite continued IL-2 administration.

IL-2/Cisplatin

Atkins et al. (1990) treated 20 patients with an IL-2/cisplatin regime. Doses of IL-2 were higher than in most other regimens here reviewed, i.e. 10^5 units/kg i.v. 8 hourly on days 1–5 and 15–19. Cisplatin was given in doses of 135–150 mg/m^2 i.v. on days 32 and 53 in conjunction with WR2721 910 mg/m^2. Nine patients received full doses of cisplatin while six had course reductions due to renal toxicity or neutropenia and five had cisplatin withheld due to persistent toxicity or progression of disease. There were three CRs and five PRs (40% overall).

Toxicity with this regime was severe and was principally due to the effects of cisplatin; ototoxicity and renal toxicity occurred in nine patients each. The use of WR2721 did not appear to protect against cisplatin toxicity in this setting.

IL-2/Interferon

Following in vitro studies of LAK cell induction which suggested a possible benefit in terms of cytotoxic action by combining interferon-α and IL-2 (Weidmann et al. 1988) there have been two preliminary reports of the combination in metastatic melanoma.

Whitehead et al. (1990) evaluated an out-patient regime of IL-2 2×10^6 units/m^2/day CI on days 1–4 each treatment week with interferon α-2a 6×10^6 units/m^2 i.m. or s.c. on days 1 and 4 of each week. Cycles were repeated two weekly. No responses were seen.

In contrast Lee et al. (1989) treated 17 patients with IL-2 3×10^6 units/m^2/day for 4 days/week and interferon α-2a 5×10^6 units/m^2/day i.m. for 4 days/week for 4 weeks. After 2–6 weeks the regime was repeated. Among 15 evaluable patients there were two PRs and one CR (20%). Chronic debilitating fatigue with weight loss resulting in a fall in performance status was dose limiting in this study.

Toxicity in these two studies has been considerable and the response data so far are a little discouraging; the objective response rate here is not better than that reported for either agent alone. Further studies are needed to establish whether the interferon/IL-2 combination in other doses or schedules has clinical advantages predicted by the work in vitro.

With all IL-2 regimes potential toxicity is a major worry. However, in our own phase II studies of 20 patients using IL-2 (3×10^6 Cetus units/m^2/24 h by CI in 5-day periods) alone or in combination with interferon-α or DTIC, toxicity was remarkably mild, though implanted i.v. line sepsis was a problem in three patients. A mild transient flu-like syndrome was invariable. Minimal hypotension was observed in 60% of patients but did not require intervention (Sheridan et al. 1991).

Summary

IL-2 biological therapy is clearly an important and exciting recent development – consistent and durable responses have been seen. Toxicity has been a major problem but lower dosage and combination regimes are now being explored to avoid this. However, there is as yet still no place for such therapy outside the clinical trial situation

Conclusion

The search for improvements in survival in metastatic malignant lymphoma continues but palliation remains the essential prerequisite for therapy. Many earlier studies reported well on response and toxicity data but did not reflect "quality of life". If we indiscriminately intensify our therapies (cytotoxic and biological), quality of life of patients must inevitably suffer. New drugs, combinations and schedules must of course be assessed, but only in properly devised studies performed in specialist treatment centres. There is clearly a need for more controlled randomized studies and there is still an ethical argument for a "symptomatically" treated control arm. However, many authorities now feel that the comparison of new treatments should be with conventional single-agent

DTIC regimes since as yet the overall advantages of combinations of cytotoxics and/or biological agents are marginal.

References

Aamdal S, Radford J, Thatcher N et al. (1990) Phase II trial of the sequential administration of DTIC and fotemustine in advanced malignant melanoma. Proc Am Assoc Cancer Res 31:200

Atkins M, Demchak P, Mier J et al. (1990) Phase II study of alternating interleukin-2 (IL-2) and cisplatin (CDDP) with WR-2721 (WR) in malignant melanoma. Proc Am Soc Clin Oncol 9:186

Avril, MF, Bonneterre J, Delaunay M et al. (1990) Combination chemotherapy of dacarbazine and fotemustine in disseminated malignant melanoma. Experience of the French Study Group. Cancer Chemother Pharmacol 27:81–84

Bajetta E, Negretti E, Giannotti B et al. (1990) Phase II study of interferon-α-2a and dacarbazine in advanced melanoma. Am J Clin Oncol 13:405–409

Balch CM, Houghton A, Peters L (1989) Cutaneous melanoma. In: De Vita V, Hellman S, Rosenberg S (eds) Cancer: principles and practice of oncology, 3rd edn, Lippincott, Philadelphia, pp 1499–1542

Bellet RE, Catalano RB, Mastrangelo MJ et al. (1978) Positive phase two trial of dibromodulcitol in patients with metastatic melanoma refractory of DTIC and nitrosourea. Cancer Treat Rep 62:2095–2099

Carmo-Pereira J, Costa OF, Hendriques E (1984) Combination cytotoxic chemotherapy with procarbazine, vincristine, and lomustine (POC) in disseminated malignant melanoma: 8 years' follow-up. Cancer Treat Rep 68:1211–1214

Chawla SP, Legha SS, Benjamin RS et al. (1985) Detrorubicin – an active anthracycline in untreated metastatic melanoma. J Clin Oncol 11:1529–1534

Cornbleet MA, McElwain TJ, Kumar PJ et al. (1983) Treatment of advanced malignant melanoma with high dose melphalan and ABMT. Br J Cancer 48:329–334

Costanza ME, Nathanson L, Schoenfeld D et al. (1977) Results with methyl-CCNU and DTIC in metastatic melanoma. Cancer 40:1010–1015

Creagan ET, Ahmann DL, Green SJ et al. (1984) Phase II study of recombinant leukocyte A interferon (r-IFN α A) in disseminated malignant melanoma. Cancer 54:2844–2849

Creagan ET, Ahmann DL, Frytak S et al. (1987) Three consecutive phase II studies of recombinant interferon alfa-2a in advanced malignant melanoma. Cancer 59:638–646

Del Prete SA, Maurer LH, O'Donnell J et al. (1984) Combination chemotherapy with cisplatin carmustine dacarbazine and tamoxifen in the treatment of malignant melanoma. Cancer Treat Rep 68:1403–1405

Dorval T, Palangie T, Jouve M et al. (1986) Clinical phase II trial of recombinant DNA interferon (interferon alfa 2b) in patients with metastatic malignant melanoma. Cancer 58:215–218

Evans BD, Hardy J, Thompson PT, Davis A, Harvey VJ (1990) A phase II study of combination chemotherapy with procarbazine, vincristine and CCNU (POC) in patients with metastatic malignant melanoma. Proc Am Soc Clin Oncol 9:276

Falkson CI, Falkson G, Falkson HC (1990) Improved results with the addition of recombinant interferon-alpha-2b to dacarbazine in treatment of patients with metastatic malignant melanoma. Proc Am Assoc Cancer Res 31:A1185

Flaherty LE, Redman BG, Chabot GG et al. (1990) A phase I–II study of dacarbazine in combination with outpatient interleukin-2 in metastatic malignant melanoma. Cancer 65:2471–2477

Gentile PS, Epremian BE, Seeger J et al. (1988) A phase II trial of vinblastine, bleomycin and cisplatin induction followed by dacarbazine and dibromodulcitol maintenance in the treatment of metastatic melanoma. A follow-up study of twenty-two patients. Am J Clin Oncol 11:666–668

Glover D, Glick JH, Weiler C et al. (1987) WR-2721 and high-dose cisplatin: an active combination in the treatment of metastatic melanoma. J Clin Oncol 5:574–578

Glover D, Grabelsky S, Fox K et al. (1989) Clinical trials of WR-2721 and cis-platinum. Int J Radiat Oncol Biol Phys 16:1201–1204

Gore M, Avril MF, O'Brean M et al. (1991) Sequential fractionated administration of low dose dacarbazine and fotemustine in disseminated malignant melanoma – preliminary results. Melanoma '91:A16

Gundersen S (1987) Dacarbazine, vindesine and cisplatin combination chemotherapy in advanced malignant melanoma: a phase II study. Cancer Treat Rep 71:997–999

Harvey H, Lipton A, Simmonds M et al. (1988) Chemotherapy (DTIC) and aromatase. Inhibition in metatstatic melanoma. Proc Am Soc Clin Oncol 7:252

Hersey P, Hasic E, MacDonald M et al. (1985) Effects of recombinant leucocyte interferon (rIFN-α-a) on tumour growth and immune responses in patients with metastatic melanoma. Br J Cancer 51:815–826

Jacquillat C, Khayat D, Banzet P et al. (1990a) Final report of the French multicenter phase II study of the nitrosourea fotemustine in 153 evaluable patients with disseminated malignant melanoma including patients with cerebral metastases. Cancer 66:1873–1878

Jacquillat C, Khayat D, Banzet P et al. (1990b) Chemotherapy by fotemustine in cerebral metastses of disseminated malignant melanoma. Cancer Chemother Pharmacol 25:263–266

Kirkwood JM, Ernstoff MS, Giuliano A et al. (1990) Interferon alpha-2a and dacarbazine in melanoma. J Natl Cancer Inst 82:1062–1063

Lakhani S, Selby P, Bliss JM et al. (1990) Chemotherapy for malignant melanoma: combinations and high doses produce more responses without survival benefit. Br J Cancer 61:330–334

Lee K, Talpaz M, Legha S et al. (1989) Combination treatment of recombinant human interleukin-2 and recombinant interferon alpha-2a in patients with advanced melanoma. Proc Am Soc Clin Oncol 8:290

Legha SS, Papadopoulos NEJ, Plager C et al. (1987) Clinical evaluation of recombinant interferon alfa-2a (Roferon-A) in metastatic melanoma using two different schedules. J Clin Oncol 5:1240–1246

Legha SS, Ring S, Papadopoulos N et al. (1989) A prospective evaluation of a triple-drug regimen containing cisplatin, vinblastine, and dacarbazine (CVD) for metastatic melanoma. Cancer 64:2024–2029

Legha S, Gianan M, Plager C et al. (1990a) Phase I–II study of IL-2 used as a continuous infusion in patients with metastatic melanoma. Proc Am Assoc Cancer Res 31:176

Legha SS, Ring S, Papadopoulos N et al. (1990b) A phase II trial of taxol in metastatic melanoma. Cancer 65:2478–2481

Margolin K, Doroshow J, Akman S et al. (1990) Treatment of advanced melanoma with CDDP and alpha interferon. Proc Am Soc Clin Oncol 9:227

McClay EF, Mastrangelo MJ (1988) Systemic chemotherpy for metastatic melanoma. Semin Oncol 15:569–577

McClay EF, Mastrangelo MJ, Bellet RE et al. (1987) Combination chemotherapy and hormonal therapy in the treatment of malignant melanoma. Cancer Treat Rep 71:465–469

McClay EF, Mastrangelo MJ, Sprandio JD et al. (1989) The importance of tamoxifen to a cisplatin-containing regimen in the treatment of metastatic melanoma. Cancer 63:1292–1295

McLeod GRC, Thomson DB, Hersey P (1987) Recombinant interferon alfa-2a in advanced malignant melanoma. A phase I–II study in combination with DTIC. Int J Cancer Suppl 1:31–35

McLeod GR, Thomson DB, Hersey P (1990) Clinical evaluation of interferons in malignant melanoma. J Invest Dermatol 95:185S–187S

Medina W, Kirkwood JM (1982) Phase II trial of mitolactol in patients with metastatic melanoma. Cancer Treat Rep 66:195–196

Mickiewicz E, Estevez R, Rao F et al. (1990) Interferon-alpha-2b (RIFN-alpha-2b) alone or in combination with DTIC in metastatic melanoma (MM). Compiled data. Proc Am Soc Clin Oncol 9:281

Mitchell MS, Kempf RA, Harel W et al. (1988) Effectiveness and tolerability of low-dose cyclophosphamide and low-dose intravenous interleukin-2 in disseminated melanoma. J Clin Oncol 6:409–424

Mortimer JE, Schulman S, MacDonald JS et al. (1990) High-dose cisplatin in disseminated melanoma: a comparison of two schedules. Cancer Chemother Pharmacol 25:373–376

Mughal TI, Robinson WA, Thomas MR et al. (1988) Role of recombinant interferon-alpha-2 in treatment of advanced malignant melanoma. Proc Am Soc Clin Oncol 7:A969

Mulder JH, Dodiodn P, Cavalli F et al. (1982) Cisplatinum and vindesine combination therapy in advanced melanoma: an EORTC phase two study. Eur J Clin Oncol 18:1297–1301

Murray N, Silver H, Shah A et al. (1985) Phase two trial of mitolactol in advanced malignant melanoma. Cancer Treat Rep 69:723–724

Neefe JR, Legha SS, Markowitz A et al. (1990) Phase II study of recombinant alpha-interferon in malignant melanoma. Am J Clin Oncol 13:472–476

Oneda JM, Nelson KK, Pilarski SM et al. (1990) Combination chemotherpy with cisplatin and nifedipine: synergistic antitumour effects against a cisplatin-resistant subline of the B16 amelanotic melanoma. Clin Exp Metastasis 8:59–73

Papadopoulos NE, Howard J, Murray JL et al. (1989) Phase II DTIC and interleukin 2 (IL-2) trial for metastatic malignant melanoma. Proc Am Soc Clin Oncol 8:277

Parkinson DR, Abrams JS, Wiernik PH et al. (1990) Interleukin-2 therapy in patients with metastatic malignant melanoma: a phase II study. J Clin Oncol 8:1650–1656

Pectasides D, Yianniotis H, Alevizakos N et al. (1989) Treatment of metastatic malignant melanoma with dacarbazine, vindesine and cisplatin. Br J Cancer 60:627–629

Peters WP, Eder JP, Henner WD et al. (1986) High-dose combination alkylating agents with autologous bone marrow support: a phase I trial. J Clin Oncol 4:646–654

Prudente Foundation Melanoma Study Group (1989) Chemotherapy of disseminated melanoma with bleomycin, vincristine, CCNU and DTIC (BOLD regimen). Cancer 63:1676–1680

Quagliana JM, Stephens RL, Baker LH, Costanzi JJ (1984) Vindesine in patients with metastatic malignant melanoma: a Southwest Oncology Group study. J Clin Oncol 2:316–319

Retsas S, Stockdale A, Nicoll J (1985) Impact of chemotherapy on survival of patients with metastatic malignant melanoma; results of 240 patients treated at the Westminster Hospital. Eur Conf Clin Oncol A235

Rosenberg S, Lotze M, Muul L et al. (1987) A progress report on the treatment of 157 patients with advanced cancer using lymphokine-activated killer cells and interleukin-2 or high-dose interleukin-2 alone. N Engl J Med 316:889–897

Rowinsky EK, Cazenave LA, Donehower RC (1990) Taxol: a novel investigational antimicrotubule agent. J Natl Cancer Inst 82:1247–1259

Santen RJ, Santner SJ, Harvey HA et al. (1988) Marked heterogeneity of aromatase activity in human malignant melanoma tissue. Eur J Cancer Clin Oncol 24:1811–1816

Schallreuter KU, Wood JM (1991) Fotemustine: a promising new drug in the treatment of malignant melanoma. Melanoma '91:A5

Schallreuter KU, Gleason FK, Wood JM (1990) The mechanism of action of the nitrosourea antitumor drugs on thioredoxin reductase, glutathione reductase and ribonucleotide reductase. Biochim Biophys Acta 1054:14–20

Seigler HF, Lucas VS Jr, Pharm BS et al. (1980) DTIC, CCNU, bleomycin and vincristine (BOLD) in metastatic melanoma. Cancer 46:2346–2348

Shelley W, Quirt I, Bodurtha A et al. (1985) Lomustine, vincristine, and procarbazine in the treatment of metastatic malignant melanoma. Cancer Treat Rep 69:941–944

Sheridan E, Screenivasan T, Dorreen MS, Rees RC, Hancock BW (1991) Clinical management of patients undergoing interleukin-2 therapy. Melanoma '91:A60

Simmonds MA, Lyston A, Harvey HA et al. (1985) Phase two study of dibromodulcitol in metastatic malignant melanoma. Cancer Treat Rep 69:65–67

Skornick Y, Topalian S, Rosenberg S (1990) Comparative studies of the long term growth of lymphocytes from tumour infiltrates, tumour draining lymph nodes and peripheral blood by repeated in vitro stimulation with autologous tumour. J Biol Response Mod 9:431–438

Stoter G, Shiloni E, Gundersen S et al. (1989) Alternating recombinant human interleukin-2 (rIL2) and dacarbazine (DTIC) in metastatic melanoma. Proc Am Soc Clin Oncol 8:281

Tchekmedyian NS, Tait N, Van Echo D et al. (1986) High-dose chemotherapy without autologous bone marrow transplantation in melanoma. J Clin Oncol 4:1811–1818

Thatcher N, Lind M, Morgenstern G et al. (1989) High-dose, double alkylating agent chemotherapy with DTIC melphalan, or ifosfamide and marrow rescue for metastatic malignant melanoma. Cancer 63:1296–1302

Thigpen T, Blessing J, Ball H et al. (1990) Phase two trial of taxol a second line therapy for ovarian cancer. A Gynaecologic oncology group study. Proc Am Soc Clin Oncol 9:604

Verschraegen CF, Kleeberg UR, Mulder J et al. (1988) Combination of cisplatin, vindesine, and dacarbazine in advanced malignant melanoma. A phase II study of the EORTC Malignant Melanoma Cooperative Group. Cancer 62:1061–1065

Vorobiof DA, Falkson G, Voges CW (1989) DTIC versus DTIC and recombinant interferon α-2b (rIFN-α-2b) in the treatment of patients (Pts) with advanced malignant melanoma. Proc Am Soc Clin Oncol 8:284

Wagner DE, Ramirez G Weiss AJ (1972) Combination phase I–II study of imidazole carboxamide. Oncology 26:310–316

Walker MJ, Beattie CW, Patel MK et al. (1987) Estrogen receptor in malignant melanoma. J Clin Oncol 5:1256–1261

Weidmann E, Bergmann L, Mitrou PS, Hoelzer D (1988) Influence of different cytokines and OKT3 antibodies on LAK cell induction in vitro. J Cancer Res Clin Oncol 41:144

West WH, Trauer KW, Schwartzenberg LS et al. (1988) Constant infusion recombinant interleukin in the treatment of advanced renal carcinoma. Proc Am Soc Clin Oncol 7:124

Whitehead RP, Kopecky KJ, Samson JJ et al. (1989) A phase II study of IV bolus recombinant interleukin-2 (IL-2) in metastatic malignant melanoma: a Southwest Oncology Group study. Proc Am Soc Clin Oncol 8:284

Whitehead RP, Figlin R, Citron ML et al. (1990) A phase II study of concomitant recombinant human interleukin-2 (IL-2) and recombinant interferon alpha-2a (alpha-IFN) in patients with disseminated malignant melanoma. Proc Am Soc Clin Oncol 9:281

Wiernik PH, Schwartz EL, Einzig A et al. (1987) Phase I trial of taxol given as a 24 hour infusion every 21 days: responses observed in metastatic melanoma. J Clin Oncol 5:1232–1239

York RM, Foltz AT (1988) Bleomycin, vincristine, lomustine and DTIC chemotherapy for metastatic melanoma. Cancer 61:2183–2186

Young DW, Lever RS, English JSC et al. (1985) The use of BELD combination chemotherapy (bleomycin, vindesine, CCNU, and DTIC) in advanced malignant melanoma. Cancer 55:1879–1881

12 Progress and Prospects for Therapeutic Targeting Strategies for Disseminated Melanoma

P. A. Riley

Introduction: The Problem of Disseminated Melanoma

At present, early detection and surgical removal offers the only adequate curative treatment for melanoma. the effectiveness of existing therapy against disseminated melanoma is inadequate and radiation therapy is generally ineffective. Most of the drugs currently used against melanoma exhibit less than 25% of responses (Lejeune 1986; Drzewiecki et al. 1990; Mulder et al. 1990). Thus improvements in the chemotherapy for patients with disseminated melanoma is an important priority.

Possible Targeting Strategies

Most of the current chemotherapy of cancer is based on selectivity which is related to inflicting damage on rapidly proliferating cells, and this depends on the generally higher proliferation rate of melanoma cells. But clearly this approach is inadequate in the treatment of disseminated melanoma in which many metastatic cells are dormant or slowly proliferating. Thus a need for novel targeting strategies is clear. The melanoma targeting strategies that are described below have been developed on the basis either of specific cell surface markers or on the pigment-generating metabolism characteristic of melanocytes (Table 12.1).

Cell Surface Molecules

This strategy is essentially based on either the recognition of cell surface molecules such as receptors for hormones or other agonists, or the detection of antigenic epitopes of surface molecules characteristic of melanoma cells. Specific

Table 12.1. Melanoma targeting strategies

Cell surface molecules
Receptors (hormones, growth factors)
Antigens
Melanogenesis
Exploitation of cytotoxic potential of natural melanogens (inhibition of protective mechanisms)
Pro-drug activation by melanogenic enzymes
Incorporation of exogenous thiols
Uptake of melanin-binding agents

binding to such cell surface markers is an obvious general strategy for targeting cytotoxic therapy in cancer. Many studies are in progress which may disclose suitable antigenic marker molecules that may provide specific targets for future treatment of melanoma.

The demonstration of specific alpha-melanocyte stimulating hormone (α-MSH) receptors on human melanoma cells (Ghanem et al. 1988; Solca et al. 1989) has prompted the development of α-MSH-linked cytotoxic targeting. Several attempts to use this receptor targeting method have been recorded in the literature. For example, α- or β-MSH fragments have been used as covalently linked carriers for various compounds, such as daunomycin (Varga et al. 1977), tobacco mosaic virus (Kriwaczek et al. 1978), ricin A chain (Griffin, et al. 1981), N-(2-boroethyl)-N-nitrosocarbamoyl (Suli-Vargha et al. 1984), ML cyclomycin (Lewensohn et al. 1985), diphtheria toxin (Murphy et al. 1986), and antibody to CD3 (Liu et al. 1988). So far one of the most promising of such MSH-linked agents is α-MSH-melphalan, and this approach is described in more detail below.

Melanogenic Pathway

The other major targeting strategy depends on utilizing the unique metabolism of melanocytes that is involved in the generation of pigment. Although some of the details of the later stages of melanogenesis remain obscure, the initial steps in the process have been well established and involve the enzymatic oxidation of tyrosine to the corresponding orthoquinone (dopaquinone) followed by a series of reactions yielding the indolic precursors of melanin (Fig. 12.1).

These reactions are normally confined to specialized organelles (melanosomes). The potential toxicity of some natural melanogens has been recognized for a considerable time (Hochstein and Cohen 1963). The presence of reactive species, such as orthoquinones and their corresponding semiquinones, among the metabolic intermediates of melanogenesis requires the process to be segregated from the cytosol (Slater and Riley 1966). An interesting recent development is the recognition that in many melanomas the limiting membrane of melanosomes is defective (Borovansky, personal communication).

Another important protective mechanism against the potential toxicity of natural melanogens is the reaction of low-molecular-weight thiols with the quinone products of tyrosine oxidation. The major reactions appear to involve either cysteine or glutathione (Fig. 12.2). The studies of Rorsman and others (see review by Karg et al. 1991) indicate that cysteine is the major reactant present

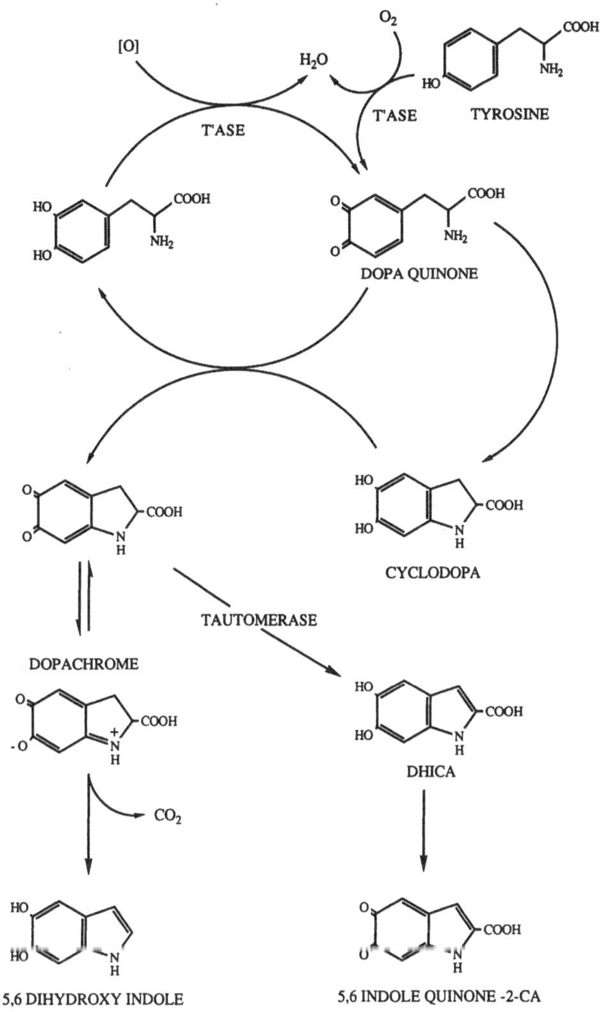

Fig. 12.1. Schematic summary of phase 1 melanogenesis. The two oxidizing actions of tyrosinase (T'ASE) are illustrated. The monophenolase activity (shown on the right) converts tyrosine into dopaquinone. The dehydrogenation reaction (shown on the left) converts catechols, in this case 3,4-dihydroxyphenylalanine (DOPA) into the corresponding quinone. Endocyclization of dopaquinone to cyclodopa is spontaneous and is rapidly followed by oxidation of cyclodopa by a redox exchange with dopaquinone to yield dopa and dopachrome. This may undergo spontaneous decarboxylation to yield 5,6-dihydroxyindole (DHI) or is acted on by dopachrome tautomerase to yield 5,6,-dihydroxyindole-2-carboxylic acid (DHICA) which is then further oxidized, probably by redox exchange with dopaquinone to form the corresponding 5,6-indole quinone-2-carboxylic acid which undergoes further reactions and polymerizes to give rise to eumelanin. The mechanisms of indole polymerization (phase 2 melangogenesis) are not fully understood.

within melanosomes. Nucleophilic addition of cysteine to dopaquinone gives rise predominantly to 5-S-cysteinyldopa and this reaction is regarded as an important branching point in the generation of phaeomelanins (Prota 1980). Reactions involving nucleophilic addition of glutathione (GSH) are apparently less significant (Karg et al. 1991) and may indicate that this constitutes a reaction which

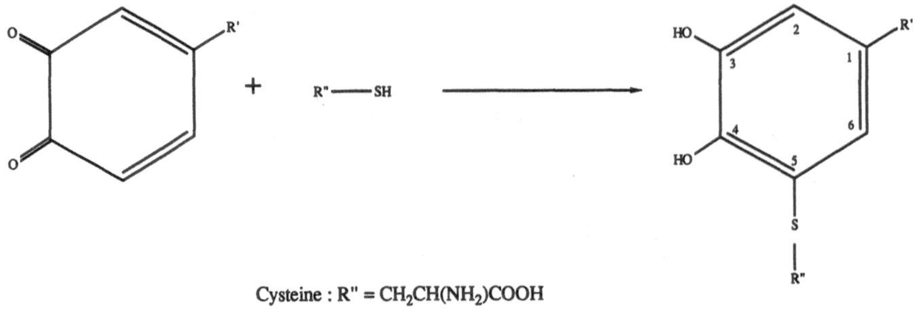

Cysteine : R" = CH$_2$CH(NH$_2$)COOH

GSH : R" = CH$_2$ CH$\begin{cases} \text{CH}_2\text{CH(NH}_2)\text{COOH} \\ \text{NHCOCH}_2\text{CH}_2\text{CH(NH}_2)\text{COOH} \end{cases}$

Fig. 12.2. Detoxification of orthoquinones. Generalized schematic outline of reductive addition of thiols to orthoquinone. Although the 5-position of the ring is favoured for the nucleophilic addition of thiols, addition at the 2 and 6 positions may also take place. Reaction with low-molecular-weight thiols is regarded as a mechanism for detoxification of orthoquinones in the cell.

takes place predominantly outside melanosomes. Thus GSH addition to ortho-quinones may represent an important protective mechanism to prevent the cytotoxic action of melanogenic products leaking from the melanosomes. Interference with this mechanism by lowering cellular GSH levels may prove to be an additional approach to melanoma therapy when used in conjunction with other methods, although studies with agents such as buthionine sulphoxine (BSO) that deplete cellular GSH levels have hitherto been disappointing.

Incorporation of extraneous low-molecular-weight thiols in the melanogenic process has been investigated in some detail, especially by the group of Larsson (see review by Larsson 1991). In particular, the method has utilized aminothiols such as thiouracil (Fig. 12.3) labelled with a gamma-emitting radionuclide as a diagnostic procedure for detection of sites of active melanogenesis. The possibility of using a short-range radioisotope for therapeutic use with such agents has been investigated using ^{35}S-labelled material. Also, recently, the feasibility of using [10]B-labelled material with subsequent neutron capture activation has been investigated. There are also possibilities of using this technique for targeting cytotoxic agents to the cell.

In addition to these reactions there are protective mechanisms connected with the inactivation of dihydroxy products generated during melanogenesis, in particular the indoles 5,6-dihydroxyindole (DHI) and 5,6-dihydroxyindole-2-carboxylic acid (DHICA). Probably the most important enzyme is catechol O-methyl transferase (COMT) which was identified in melanocytes by Pavel et al. (1983). This enzyme appears to be located largely in the cytosol and by methylation prevents the further oxidation of dihydroxy intermediates of mela-nogenesis (Fig. 12.4). The methylated compounds are excreted and thus provide a means of monitoring melanogenesis and therefore the possibility for use in diagnosis or monitoring therapy. There is evidence that the auto-oxidation of catechols generates reactive oxygen species (ROS), especially hydrogen perox-ide, which are cytotoxic. Thus, inhibition of COMT might prove to be therapeuti-cally beneficial in melanoma.

The possibility of amplifying the potential toxicity of melanogenesis by

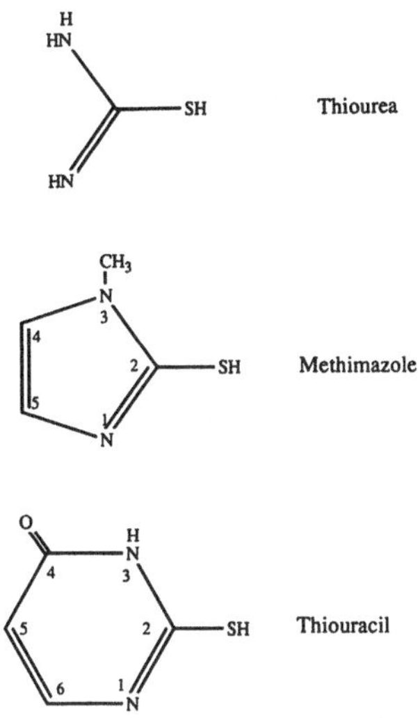

Fig. 12.3. Thiourea derivatives that are incorporated into nascent melanin by reaction with quinone intermediates. The mechanism of incorporation appears to involve reductive addition of the kind illustrated in Fig. 12.2.

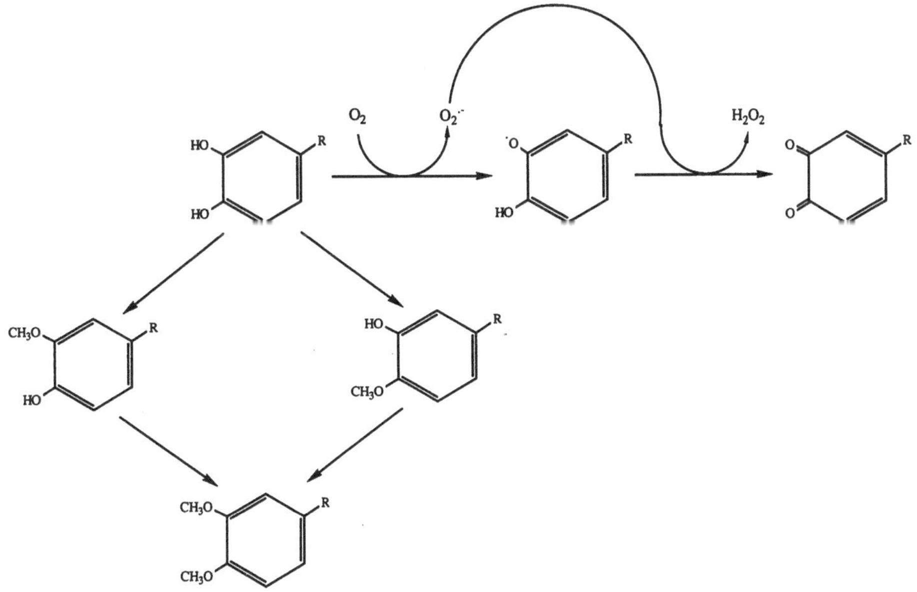

Fig. 12.4. Detoxification of catechols. The figure schematically illustrates the tendency for catecholic substances to undergo auto-oxidation and generate reactive oxygen species such as superoxide and H_2O_2. This potentially toxic reaction pathway is abrogated by methylation of the hydroxyl groups either in the 3 or the 4 position of the ring giving rise to monomethoxycatechols, or if both hydroxyl groups are methylated to the dimethoxy product. The methoxy products are inhibited from undergoing auto-oxidation.

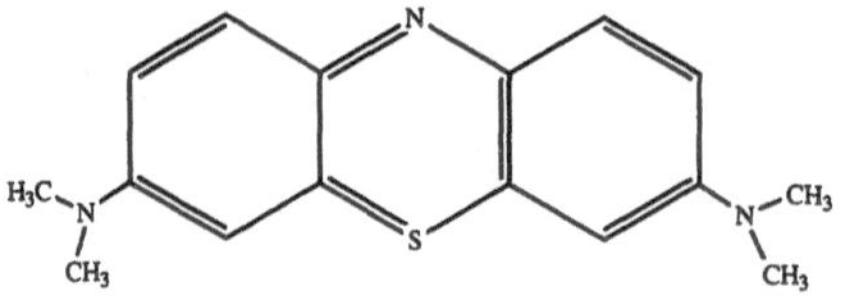

Fig. 12.5. The structure of methylene blue.

diversion of the intermediate oxidative products was suggested by the discovery that the mode of action of a class of phenolic depigmenting agents was related to their ability to act as alternative substrates for tyrosinase catalysed oxidation (Riley 1969). Oxidation of these phenols gives rise to reactive orthoquinones which become diverted from the normal melanogenic pathway. The nature of the cytotoxic mechanism remains to be fully elucidated but appears to depend on the relative stability of the orthoquinones generated from the analogue substrates which results from the absence of an endocyclizing side chain. Such quinones are more likely to penetrate the melanosomal membrane and initiate toxic damage in melanocytes. The mechanism of cytotoxicity has been ascribed to the generation of reactive oxygen species by redox cycling, or by the initiation of lipid peroxidation by the semiquinone radicals that are known to be formed as the result of oxidation of these analogue substrates (Riley 1985). However, recent evidence (Land et al. 1990) suggests that the mechanism involves the reaction of the orthoquinones with crucial protein thiols in the cell. A range of tyrosine analogues has been investigated for potential antimelanoma activity and one compound, 4-hydroxyanisole (4HA), has been used in pilot clinical studies with some promising results.

The possibility of using melanin-binding agents as a method for selective delivery of cytotoxic drugs or radionuclides has also been investigated. This method, although less selective with regard to the origin of the pigment to which it binds, has been developed mainly in relation to the binding of phenothiazines (Fig. 12.5) to preformed melanin. This process appears to be brought about by the formation of a charge-transfer complex and it has long been known that phenothiazine derivatives bind strongly to melanin. Recently it has been shown (Link and Carpenter 1990) that methylene blue (MTB), which is essentially non-toxic but binds strongly to melanin, has a strong therapeutic action on melanoma when labelled with the short-range alpha particle emitter[211]At.

Experimental Targeted Antimelanoma Therapy

Receptor-Linked Cyotoxicity Using α-MSH

Although α-MSH receptors are apparently not present on normal human melanocytes, they have been demonstrated on human melanoma cells (Ghanem et al. 1988). It is known that these receptors are internalized and possess a rapid turnover (Varga et al. 1976; Orlow et al. 1990) and on the basis of these

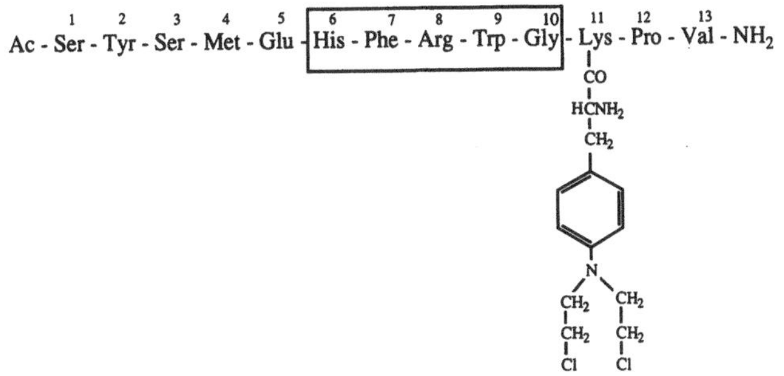

Fig. 12.6. The structure of the α-MSH–melphalan complex. Melphalan is covalently attached to the lysyl residue in position 11 of the peptide. The boxed area represents the receptor recognition sequence of α-MSH.

observations melanoma targeting using α-MSH as a drug carrier has been investigated, using α-MSH coupled to melphalan (Fig. 12.6). Melphalan is a powerful and well-known alkylating agent. It was linked to α-MSH at the lysine residue in position 11 of α-MSH. This amino acid is not contained in the main receptor recognition region of α-MSH (Eberle et al. 1977). Binding assays have shown that the MSH-melphalan complex exhibits increased binding efficiency to the receptor, but this may be due to alkylation of membrane components. Using material iodinated with ^{125}I Ghanem et al. (1991) have shown rapid tissue distribution of the material and specific binding to melanoma tissue in experimental animals. In vitro cytotoxicity tests have shown that the degree of cytotoxicity is closely related to the α-MSH receptor density found on various human melanoma cell lines. Comparison of the cytotoxicity of α-MSH-melphalan showed up to two orders of magnitude greater toxicity compared with melphalan alone. Moreover, cell lines with low MSH receptor density were found to be no more sensitive to the α-MSH–melphalan complex than to melphalan alone. Thus, the in vitro data for this targeting strategy are very encouraging.

Melanogenesis

The characteristic and unique metabolic pathway present in melanocytes, and to a greater or lesser extent in melanoma cells, is the melanogenic pathway. As a targeting strategy it seems rational to attempt to subvert the natural melanogenic mechanism to generate toxic compounds from innocuous pro-drugs. In addition, as outlined above, the process of melanogenesis involves the generation of potentially toxic intermediates and the cells possess protective mechanisms to reduce the likelihood of autotoxicity by this metabolic process. The three protective mechanisms identified include the following:

1. The interposition of a membrane between the melanogenic organelle and the rest of the cytosol
2. Reaction of quinones with thiols
3. *O*-methylation of dihydroxy-compounds

It is possible that by specific interference with the normal protein targeting of tyrosinase damage could be induced in the affected cells. However, currently there do not seem to be any obvious possibilities for the development of such an approach, or one that involves interference with the lipid membrane surrounding melanosomes without causing general toxicity to the organism.

Incorporation of Extraneous Thiols

The reactivity of the intermediate orthoquinones of melanogenesis with low-molecular-weight thiols offers a means of developing a melanoma-seeking drug. Selective uptake of thiouracil by melanogenic tissue was first demonstrated by Whittaker (1971). Dencker et al. (1979) showed that 2-thiouracil accumulates in sites of rapid melanogenesis and it has also been shown that thiouracil is not bound to preformed melanin (Dencker et al. 1981). Uptake of radioactively labelled thiouracil was found to be located in melanotic melanomas in experimental animals but was not localized in amelanotic melanomas (Dencker et al. 1982). These findings have been confirmed by several laboratories (Fairchild et al. 1982; Levine et al. 1983) and the chemical mechanism involved in the uptake of 2-thiouracil has been elucidated (Palumbo et al. 1990).

The diagnostic possibilities of this specific uptake have been examined using 5-iodo-2-thiouracil (ITU) labelled with a gamma-emitting isotope of iodine (Larsson et al. 1982; van Langevelde et al. 1983). Radioiodinated ITU is accumulated and retained in the melanin of melanotic melanomas transplanted into mice and is also selectively localized in melanotic metastases. Pretreatment of melanoma-bearing mice with thyroxine and potassium iodide prevented accumulation of radioactivity in the thyroid of animals treated with ITU (Larsson et al. 1982). Clinically, [^{123}I]ITU has been used for diagnosis of ocular melanoma (Franken et al. 1986) and [^{131}I]ITU has been used in gamma-scintigraphy of skin melanoma patients (Olander et al. personal communication). From the therapeutic point of view, the possibility of using thioureas as selective melanoma seekers to carry locally destructive radiation to the tumour has been investigated using [^{35}S]thiouracil (Fairchild et al. 1989). In these experiments mice bearing Harding–Passey melanomas exposed to doses of radiation up to 370 MBq demonstrated complete tumour regression at the highest dose. However, apart from the very high radiation doses involved, there is a problem created by the metabolic release of ^{35}S which appears to be concentrated in cartilage. Iodine-131 may be a better choice of radionuclide for therapeutic purposes.

The possibility of using 2-thiouracil or similar compounds as carriers for cytotoxic agents has also been investigated in vitro. Watjen et al. (1982) investigated 2-thiouracil substituted in the 5-position with carotenoids and retinoids. They were able to show that the compounds were localized in melanomas but no cytostatic effect on Cloudman S-91 cells in vitro was observed. A similar lack of cytotoxic activity was found with 2-thiouracil substituted at the 5-position with nitrogen mustard when given to mice transplanted with Harding–Passey melanoma (Larsson, personal communication). This may indicate a failure of release of the alkylating agent from the complex after incorporation into melanin or its inability to diffuse to reach sensitive cellular targets.

Recent interest in boron neutron capture therapy (BNCT) has suggested the possibility of using thiourea derivatives substituted with ^{10}B which can be activated in situ by exposure to external radiation with thermal neutrons. Boron-

10 is a stable nuclide which has a large cross-section for neutron absorption and generates an alpha particle and a lithium ion on capture of a neutron:

$$^{10}B + n \rightarrow {}^{7}Li + \alpha$$

The principle of BNCT is based on irradiation of tumours with low-energy neutrons (Fairchild and Bond 1985) after accumulation of boron in the tumour and its metabolic clearance from the surrounding normal tissue. The emitted particles have high linear energy transfer over track lengths which are less than a cell diameter. A pilot clinical trial using BCNT for the treatment of melanoma was undertaken by Mishima et al. (1989) using ^{10}B-labelled phenylalanine as the tumour-locating agent. Although this procedure appears to have been successful, there are reasons to believe that thiourea would be more effective as a melanoma-localizing compound. A number of boronated thioureas have been synthesized and the uptake and distribution has been investigated by boron neutron capture radiography (Larsson 1986). Studies with the ^{10}B-adduct of 1,2,4-triazole-3-thiol have shown good incorporation into murine melanoma in vivo (Larsson et al. 1989). Although this approach holds some promise, problems remain with regard to the heterogeneous distribution of the ^{10}B in the tumours and the more general problem of the need for whole-body neutron irradiation if the procedure is to be used as a general treatment for disseminated melanoma.

Inhibition of Cytoprotective Mechanisms in Melanogenic Cells

An important mechanism for the protection of cells to reactive intermediates of the melanogenic pathway is one involving the O-methylation of the o-dihydroxy-phenolic and indolic compounds. The protective role of O-methylation in melanocytes was identified by Pavel et al. (1983) who showed that in human melanoma cell cultures the enzyme responsible for O-methylation of the o-dihydroxyindolic compounds was catechol O-methyl transferase (COMT) (Smit et al. 1990). This enzyme has been shown to have a higher affinity for 5,6-dihydroxyindole-2-carboxylic acid than the COMT of hepatic origin. There is evidence that COMT from melanotic cells is present in the cytoplasm with some of the activity located in the endoplasmic reticulum. This appears to be entirely analogous to the localization of COMT in other cells where presumably the enzyme performs a similar protective function. However, comparison of COMT activity in subcellular fractions of melanotic and amelanotic hamster melanoma cells indicates that COMT activity may be reduced in pigment-generating tumours (Shibata et al. personal communication). Since COMT is extra-melanosomal, it is unlikely that the activity of this enzyme is involved in the regulation of melanogenesis, but, on the other hand, COMT activity may be influenced by reaction with the intermediates that are generated in cells of different melanogenic potential. There is some evidence that COMT is inhibited by reaction with 5,6-dihydroxyindole which is thought to be a minor autoxidation product of the normal melanogenic pathway. In terms of a targeting strategy in melanoma treatment it may be that cells can be rendered more susceptible to the reactive intermediates generated during normal melanogenesis by inhibition of melanocytic COMT. Investigations are in progress to identify potential COMT inhibitors that distinguish between the melanoma-associated enzyme and that present in the liver.

Targeting by Melanin-Binding Agents

Many melanomas are heavily pigmented and although the degree of pigmentation may differ, especially among metastases, there is rarely a total absence of pigment. One of the reasons for the heavy pigmentation of melanomas appears to be lack of melanin transfer to other cells – a process which occurs under normal circumstances. By virtue of its relatively stable localization in melanoma cells, melanin therefore constitutes a suitable target for a melanoma-localizing agent. It is known that a range of compounds, of which the phenothiazine derivatives are of a special significance, exhibit strong binding to melanin (Potts 1964). Of these methylene blue (MTB) is of particular interest since it is relatively non-toxic but exhibits strong melanin-binding properties. Highly selective uptake of MTB has been demonstrated in pigmented melanomas in vitro and in vivo (Link and Lukiewicz 1982; Link et al. 1989). Thus, the potential of methylene blue as a carrier for cytotoxic agents or a suitable radionuclide is clear. Initial studies made with ^{35}S-labelled MTB have revealed a significant dose-dependent therapeutic advantage in vitro and in melanoma-bearing animal model systems (Link and Lukiewicz 1982). ^{35}S-labelled MTB produced significant retardation in the growth of transplanted pigmented melanomas in hamsters, both when the tumour cells were exposed to ^{35}S-labelled MTB prior to inoculation, or when the drug was administered intracutaneously close to previously established tumour sites. More recently, [211]At-labelled MTB has been used with promising results and this radionuclide carrier may prove to be suitable for targeted in situ radiotherapy of disseminated melanoma. [211]At-labelled MTB was found to be more effective by two orders of magnitude than the equivalent [35]S- and ^{125}I-analogues (Link and Carpenter 1990). It was found to be especially effective against single melanoma cells in the circulation as determined by tests using assays of metastatic potential after intravenous injection of human melanoma cells, or by inhibition of lymph node metastases derived from subcutaneously implanted human melanoma xenografts (Link and Carpenter 1991). The exceptionally short range of the energy emission from [211]At and the short half-life of this isotope render it attractive as a radionuclide for selective internal application. Clearly the radiolabelled methylene blue method may also be employed as a tumour-localizing procedure for diagnostic purposes by substitution of a gamma-emitting radionuclide.

Diversion of Melanogenesis Using Alternative Substrates for Tyrosinase

Tyrosinase is an unusual enzyme which possesses two separate activities, one of which involves ortho-hydroxylation of phenols, the so-called "monophenolase" activity, and the other is the dehydrogenation of the corresponding dihydroxyphenols to form orthoquinones. The natural substrate in eukaryotes appears to be L-tyrosine which is converted into the orthoquinone of dopa (dopaquinone). Dopaquinone acts as the major oxidizing species in the melanogenic pathway and undergoes redox exchange reactions with some of the later products in the metabolic sequence, generating 3,4-dihydroxyphenylalanine (dopa) (Fig. 12.1). Tyrosinase is a copper enzyme and the copper must be in reduced form in order for the enzyme to bind oxygen and catalyse the hydroxylation of phenols. However, the redox state of the metal is not crucial to the dehydrogenation of catechols and under most conditions, dopa is more rapidly oxidized than tyrosine. Consequently, a number of cytotoxic strategies have been investigated using catechol derivatives (e.g. Wick 1980). There is now considerable evidence that the cytotoxic effect of catechols is very largely the result of auto-oxidation of these compounds with the generation of reactive oxygen species, in particular, hydrogen peroxide, and the cytotoxicity of these compounds can be abrogated by catalase (Karg et al. 1991). In addition there are problems posed by the primary toxicity and pharmacological activity of catechols.

On the other hand, although there are some problems outstanding with regard to the primary toxicity of phenols, and in particular, the cytotoxic effects of hepatic metabolites of these compounds, the generation of potentially cytotoxic orthoquinones from phenolic substrates by tyrosinase oxidation appears to be a promising approach to specific melanocyte toxicity by diversion of the melanogenic pathway (Riley 1985). Several phenolic compounds have been studied from this point of view. In particular, a series of *para*-oxyethers and thioethers of phenol have been investigated in which a number of side-group substitutions have been made (Fig. 12.7). Recently there have also been studies on *N*-substituted phenols (Fig. 12.7), based on the structure of *N*-phenylglycine (Prota, personal communication). Although many of these reagents show highly promising tyrosinase-dependent cytotoxicity in vitro, few of them have so far been carefully examined in tumour model systems in vivo or used in the clinic. Jimbow and colleagues (Alena et al. 1990) have shown that 4-*S*-aminophenol derivatives have marked selective depigmenting action due to specific cytotoxicity to melanocytes in hair follicles of black mice. Moreover, they have shown specific cytotoxic effects on implanted melanotic tumours in animals. Of the oxyethers of phenol

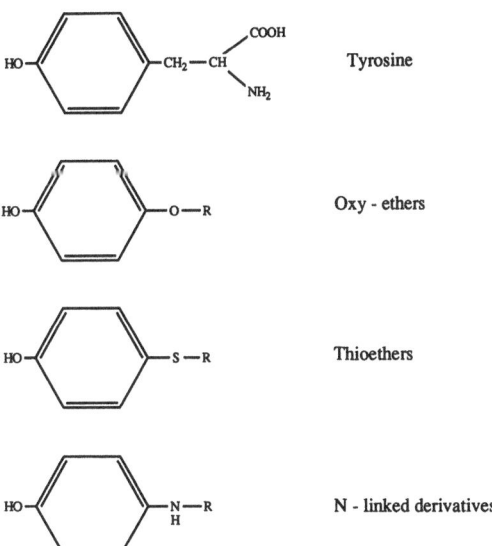

Fig. 12.7. The general structure of tyrosine analogues compared with the natural substrate of tyrosinase (L-tyrosine). A large number of alternative side-chains (represented by R) have been investigated by several laboratories. The most promising compounds to have been examined in detail for their antimelanoma activity are the oxy-ether, 4-hydroxyanisole (where R = CH_3) and the thio-ether, *N*-acetyl-4-*S*-cysteinylaminophenol (in which R = $CH_2CH(COOH)NHCOCH_3$).

that have been examined, the most studied example is that of 4-hydroxyanisole (4HA). This material has a powerful tyrosinase-dependent cytotoxicity in vitro which is related to the generation of the corresponding orthoquinone (Naish et al.

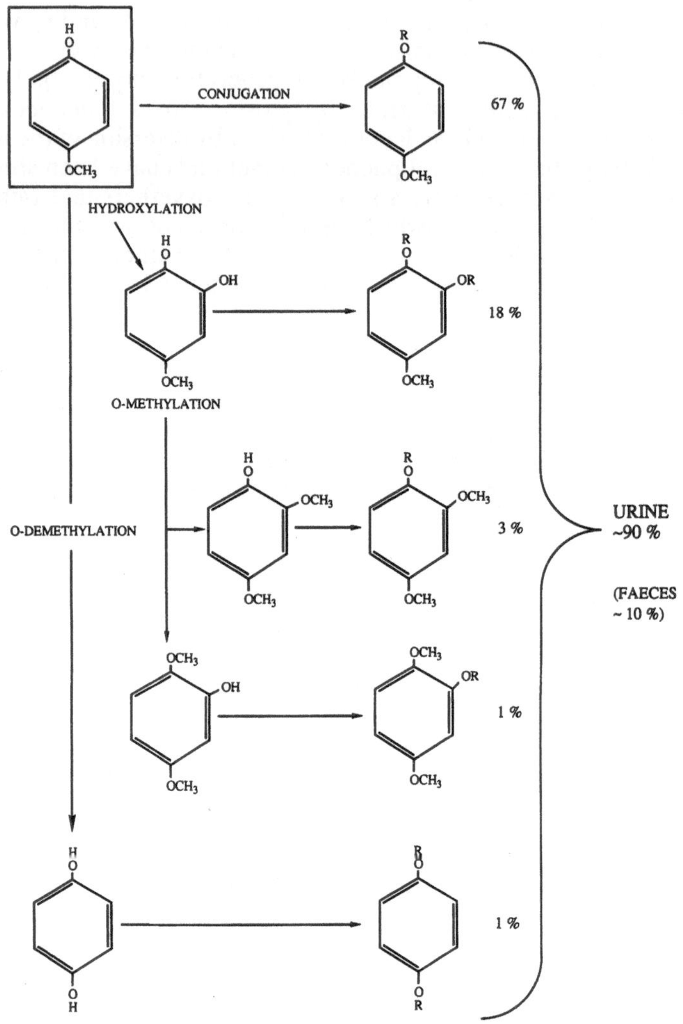

Fig. 12.8. Schematic summary of hepatic metabolism of 4HA based on metabolic products detected in the urine. The data are derived from Pavel et al. (1989). The excretory products are in a conjugated form where R = sulphate or glucuronide. O-demethylation accounts for about 1% of the total whereas over 60% of the material is excreted as the conjugated phenol. Approximately 20% of 4HA is hydroxylated to form the 3,4-dihydroxyanisole, most of which is excreted in a conjugated catecholic form. O-methylation accounts for about a quarter of the dihydroxy compound and the majority of the material is methylated in the 3 position prior to excretion. Most of the excretion (> 90%) is in the urine although other studies have shown some recovery of labelled material from the faeces.

1988). The cytotoxic action of the orthoquinone is probably due to the formation of a covalent adduct with thiol residues in important cellular proteins. There are a number of thiol-containing proteins which are of crucial importance to cellular survival, including membrane ion pumps and enzymes involved in other crucial aspects of cellular metabolism including DNA synthesis. There is also the possibility of the generation of novel antigens with the phenol acting as a hapten and this may account for the delayed responses to 4HA that have been observed (Morgan, personal communication). Although some of the S-phase specific toxicity ascribed to 4HA (Galpine and Dewey 1984) may be due to a direct action of the agent as an inhibitor of ribonucleotide reductase (Lassman et al. 1991), it is possible that some of the S-phase specific action is the result of interference with DNA synthesis due to inhibition of DNA polymerase by the corresponding orthoquinone. 4HA has been used in clinical pilot studies with promising results (Morgan et al. 1981; Morgan 1984). Responses have been observed mainly in cases treated for recurrent melanoma of the lower limb where the drug has been given by intra-arterial infusion (Morgan 1984). This, of course, limits the possibility of treatment of widely disseminated metastases and, unfortunately, the pharmacokinetics and systemic toxicity of 4HA does not permit adequate therapeutic concentrations to be achieved by intravenous administration, without the risk of serious hepatic or renal toxicity (Rustin, personal communication). The metabolic pathway of elimination of 4HA has been delineated by Pavel et al. (1989). Approximately 20% of the drug is detoxified by the liver through the intermediate generation of the 3,4-dihyroxy-species (Fig. 12.8) This material is presumably generated by P450 metabolism and is potentially toxic through its auto-oxidation products. Thus, although the subversion of melanogenesis to generate toxic species from tyrosine analogues is a promising rational approach to the chemotherapy of melanoma, there remain many serious obstacles to the optimization of this approach. This will depend on the emergence of structural analogues that are devoid of significant tyrosinase-independent toxicity and several laboratories are currently engaged in pursuit of this goal.

Conclusion

It is clear from the above that several new rational methods are being developed for selective antimelanoma treatment. Most of the methodologies are subject to difficulties and none of these potential chemotherapeutic approaches have yet been introduced into routine clinical practice. Nevertheless, the current intensification of interest in this approach and the possibility of developing not only novel agents, but also new combination therapies based on improved knowledge of the chemistry of melanogenesis holds promise for the future.

Acknowledgements.   I am grateful to Dr G. Ghanem, Professor B.S. Larsson, Dr E.M. Link and Dr S. Pavel for help in the preparation of this Chapter, and to Dr S. Naish-Byfield for drawing the figures. I am indebted to Miss Maruschka Malacos for patiently typing the manuscript.

References

Alena F, Jimbow K, Ito S (1990) Melanocytotoxicity and antimelanoma effects of phenolic amine compounds in mice in vivo. Cancer Res 50:3743–3747

Dencker L, Larsson B, Olander K, Ullberg S, Yokota M (1979) False precursors of melanin as selective melanoma seekers. Br J Cancer 39:449–452

Dencker L, Larsson B, Olander K (1981) Incorporation of thiouracil and some related compounds into growing melanin. Acta Pharmacol Toxicol 49:141–149

Dencker L, Larrson B, Olander K, Ullberg S (1982) A new melanoma seeker for possible clinical use: selective accumulation of radiolabelled thiouracil. Br J Cancer 45:95–104

Drzewiecki KT, Frydman H, Krag H, Anderson P (1990) Malignant melanoma: changing trends in factors influencing metastasis free survival from 1964–1982. Cancer 65:362–365

Eberle A, Kriwaczek VM, Schwyzer R (1977) Hormone–receptor interactions: melanotropic activities of covalent serum albumin complexes with α-melanotropin, α-melanotropin fragments and enkephalin. FEBS Lett 80:246–250

Fairchild RG, Bond VP (1985) Current status of ^{10}B-neutron capture therapy: enhancement of tumor dose via beam filtration and dose rate, and the effects of these parameters on minimum boron content: a theoretical evaluation. Int J Radiat Oncol Biol Phys 11:831–840

Fairchild RG, Packer S, Greenberg D et al. (1982) Thiouracil distribution in mice carrying transplantable melanoma. Cancer Res 42:5126–5132

Fairchild RG, Coderre JA, Packer S, Greenberg D, Laster BH (1989) Therapeutic effects of S-35-thiouracil in BALB/c mice carrying Harding–Passey melanoma. Int J Radiat Oncol Biol Phys 17:337–343

Franken NAP, van Delft JL, van Langevelde A et al. (1986) Scintimetric detection of choroidal malignant melanoma with (^{123}I)-5-iodo-2-thiouracil. Ophthalmologia 193:248–254

Galpine AR, Dewey DL (1984) Inhibition of DNA Synthesis and S-phase killing by 4-hydroxyanisole. In: Riley PA (ed.) Hydroxyanisole: recent advances in anti-melanoma therapy. IRL Press, Oxford, pp 119–127

Ghanem G, Comunale J, Libert A, Vercammen A, Lejeune F (1988) Evidence for alpha-melanocyte stimulating hormone (alpha-MSH) receptors on human malignant melanoma cells. Int J Cancer 41:248–255

Ghanem GE, Libert A, Arnold R, Vercammen A, Lejeune F (1991) Human melanoma: targeting with α-MSH melphalan conjugate. Melanoma Res 1:105–114

Griffin TW, Demartino JA, Greene HL (1981) Inhibition of leucine incorporation in cultured melanoma cells by a conjugate of melanotropin and the toxic A chain of ricin. Proc Am Assoc Cancer Res 22:212

Hochstein P, Cohen G (1963) The cytotoxicity of melanin precursors. Ann NY Acad Sci 100:876–886

Karg E, Odh G, Rosengren E, Wittbjer A, Rorsman H (1991) Melanin related biochemistry of IGR 1 human melanoma cells. Melanoma Res 1:5–14

Kriwaczek VM, Eberle AN, Muller M, Schwyzer R (1978) Tobacco mosaic virus as a carrier for small molecules. I. The preparation and characterization of a TMV/α-melanotropin conjugate. Helv Chim Acta 61:1232–1240

Land EJ, Cooksey CJ, Riley PA (1990) Reaction kinetics of 4-methoxyorthobenzoquinone in relation to its mechanism of cytotoxicity: a pulse radiolysis study. Biochem Pharmacol 39:1133–1135

Larsson BS (1986) Boron neutron capture radiography – perspectives in melanoma therapy. J Med Sci 91:263–268

Larsson BS (1991) Melanin-affinic thioureas as selective melanoma seekers. Melanoma Res 1:95–103

Larsson B, Olander K, Dencker L, Holmqvist L (1982) Accumulation of ^{125}I-labelled thiouracil and propylthiouracil in murine melanotic melanomas. Br J Cancer 46:538–550

Larsson BS, Larsson B, Roberto A (1989) Boron neutron capture therapy for malignant melanoma: an experimental approach. Pigment Cell Res 2:356–360

Lassman G, Liermann B, Arnold W, Schwabe K (1991) Ribonucleotide reductase in melanoma tissue: EPR detection in human amelanotic melanoma and quenching of the tyrosine radical by 4-hydroxyanisole. J Cancer Res Clin Oncol 117:91–95

Lejeune F (1986) Malignant melanoma. In: Slevin ML, Staquet MJ (eds) Randomized trials in cancer. A critical review by sites. Monograph Series of the EORTC, 15. Raven Press, New York, pp 549–568

Levine N, Queen L, Chalom A (1983) Detection of melanomas. Arch Dermatol 119:295–299

Lewensohn R, Hansson J, Ringborg U (1985) A peptide containing M-L-sarcolysine with preferential toxicity to a human melanoma cell line as compared to human lymphoblasts. Proc. Third European Conference on Clinical Oncology and Cancer Nursing. Stockholm, Sweden, p 79

Link EM, Carpenter RN (1990) [211]At-methylene blue for targeted radiotherapy of human melanoma xenografts: treatment of micrometastases. Cancer Res 50:2963–2967

Link EM, Carpenter RN (1991) [211]At-methylene blue for targeted radiotherapy of human melanoma xenografts: treatment of cutaneous tumours and lymph node metastases, Cancer Res (in press)

Link EM, Lukiewicz S (1982) A new radioactive drug selectively accumulating in melanoma cells. Eur J Nucl Med 7:469–473

Link EM, Brown I, Carpenter RN, Mitchell JS (1989) Uptake and therapeutic effectiveness of [125]I- and [211]At-methylene blue for pigmented melanoma in an animal model system. Cancer Res 49:4332–4337

Liu MA, Nussbaum SR, Eisen HN (1988) Hormone conjugated with antibody to CD3 mediates cytotoxic T cell lysis of human melanoma cells. Science 239:395–397

Mishima Y, Ichihashi M, Hatta S, Honda C, Yamamura K, Nakagawa T (1989) New thermal neutron capture therapy for malignant melanoma: melanogenesis-seeking ^{10}B molecule–melanoma cell interaction from in vitro to first clinical trial. Pigment Cell Res 2:226–234

Morgan BDG (1984) Recent results of a clinical pilot study of intra-arterial 4-HA chemotherapy in malignant melanoma. In: Riley PA (ed.) Hydroxyanisole: recent advances in anti-melanoma therapy. IRL Press, Oxford, pp 233–241

Morgan BDG, O'Neill T, Dewey DL, Galpine AR, Riley PA (1981) Treatment of malignant melanoma by intravascular 4-hydroxyanisole. Clin Oncol 7:227–234

Mulder NH, Sleijfer DT, De Vries EG, Schraffordt-Koops H, Willems EPH (1990) Phase II study of carboplatin and cytosine arabinoside in patients with disseminated malignant melanoma. J Cancer Res Clin Oncol 116:301–302

Murphy JR, Bishai W, Borowski M, Miyanohara A, Boyd J, Nagle S (1986) Genetic construction, expression, and melanoma-selective cytotoxicity of a diphtheria toxin-related alpha-melanocyte-stimulating hormone fusion protein. Proc Natl Acad Sci USA 83:8258–8262

Naish S, Holden JL, Cooksey CJ, Riley PA (1988) The major primary cytotoxic product of 4-hydroxyanisole oxidation by tyrosinase is 4-methoxy-orthobenzo-quinone. Pigment Cell Res, 1:382–385

Orlow SJ, Hotchkiss S, Pawelek JM (1990) Internal binding sites for MSH: analyses in wild-type and variant Cloudman melanoma cells. J Cell Physiol 142:129–136

Palumbo A, d'Ischia M, Misuraca G, Ionnone A, Prota G (1990) Selective uptake of 2-thiouracil into melanin-producing systems depends on chemical binding to enzymically generated dopaquinone. Biochim Biophys Acta 1036:221–227

Pavel S, Muskiet FAJ, De Ley L, The TH, Van der Slik W (1983) Identification of three indolic compounds in a pigmented melanoma cell-culture supernatant by gas chromatography–mass spectrometry. J Cancer Res Clin Oncol 105:275–279

Pavel S, Holden JL, Riley PA (1989) The metabolism of 4-hydroxyanisole: identification of major urinary excretory products. Pigment Cell Res 2:421–426

Potts AM (1964) The reaction of uveal pigment in vitro with polycyclic compounds. Invest. Ophthalmol 3:405–416

Prota G (1980) Recent advances in the chemistry of melanogenesis in mammals. J Invest Dermatol 75:122–127

Riley PA (1969) Hydroxyanisole depigmentation: in vitro studies. J Pathol 97:193–206

Riley PA (1985) Radicals and melanoma. Phil Trans R Soc Lond B 311:679–689

Slater TF, Riley PA (1966) Photosensitization and lysosomal damage. Nature 209:151–153

Smit N, Pavel S, Kammeyer A, Westerhof W (1990) Determination of catechol-O-methyltransferase in relation to melanin metabolism with high-performance liquid chromatography with fluorimetric detection. Anal Biochem 190:286–291

Solca F, Siegrist W, Drozdz R, Girard J, Eberle AN (1989) The receptor for α-melanotropin of mouse and human melanoma. Application of a potent α-melanotropin photoaffinity label. J Biol Chem 264:14277–14281

Suli-Vargha H, Medzihradszky K (1984) Synthesis of N-(2-chloroethyl)-N-nitrosocarbamoyl derivatives of biologically active polypeptide hormone fragments. Int J Peptide Protein Res 23:650–656

van Langevelde A, Bakker CNM, Broxterman HJ et al. (1983) Potential radiopharmaceuticals for the detection of ocular melanoma. Part I. 5-Iodo-2-thiouracil derivatives. Eur J Nucl Med 8:45–51

Varga JM, Moellman G, Fritsch P, Godawska E (1976) Association of cell surface receptors for melanotropin with the Golgi region in mouse melanoma cells. Proc Natl Acad Sci USA 73:559–562

Varga JM, Asato N, Lande S, Lerner AB (1977) Melanotropin daunomycin conjugate shows receptor mediated cytotoxicity in cultured murine melanoma cells. Nature 267:56–58

Watjen F, Buchardt O, Langvad E (1982) Affinity therapeutics. 1. Selective incorporation of 2-thiouracil derivatives in murine melanomas. Cytostatic activity of 2-thiouracil carotinoids, and retinoids. J Med Chem 25:956–960

Whittaker JR (1971) Biosynthesis of a thiouracil pheomelanin in embryonic pigment cells exposed to thiouracil. J Biol Chem 246:6217–6226

Wick MM (1980) An experimental approach to the chemotherapy of melanoma. J Invest Dermatol 74:63–65

13 Psychological Aspects of Malignant Melanoma

Lesley Fallowfield

You just never believe that these things are going to happen to you – other people maybe, but not you. It was very easy to forget about it and pretend that it wasn't there and work always kept me so busy, as you know, so I just kept putting it off. Even after the biopsy, still I thought that I might just get away with it, but I can't say that I really thought about it much – you know me, I don't look for trouble. I'm not really sad for me, just everyone else. You've all got to be brave and remember that I'm so lucky and happy to be surrounded by so much love. That matters more – having such marvellous friends matters more than anything else.

(BM 1990)

A diagnosis of cancer and its treatment can create considerable distress, anxiety and depression, together with social, occupational and sexual dysfunction for both patients and their families. The abundant anecdotal material available in the lay, nursing and medical press which revealed this psychosocial trauma has now been reinforced and substantiated by an increasing number of studies published in the scientific literature. This research, using standardized assessments, has provided a much clearer picture of the primary areas of concern for patients at different stages of disease and treatment. The research also permits us to evaluate the impact of various interventions such as counselling and psychotherapy which aim to prevent or alleviate some of the distress. Between 25% and 35% of patients, irrespective of the site of their cancer, experience serious psychiatric morbidity that is unremitting without help and merits psychiatric intervention. However, many patients do adjust well and may express very positive attitudes to life. Even those individuals with a poor prognosis may comment that the experience of cancer has provided them with an enhanced view and appreciation of the value of life. This may be especially true as far as their relationships with family and friends are concerned. The benefits of good social support are clearly demonstrated in the quotation above taken from a discussion with a 43-year-old man dying from malignant melanoma.

Doctors who understand the potential psychosocial problems that their patients may develop and the way in which different individuals cope with the existential crisis of cancer, can do much to prevent or ameliorate psychological trauma. They can also improve the quality if not the quantity of their patients' lives through good communication and counselling skills.

Psychosocial Problems

Successful psychosocial adaptation demands that an individual develops and utilizes appropriate strategies for dealing with the problems surrounding (a) the knowledge of having a life-threatening disease, and (b) the side effects of treatment for cancer. The potential problems that are experienced by cancer patients in general are summarized in Table 13.1 and those areas of concern particularly relevant to melanoma patients will be elaborated further.

Table 13.1. Problems experienced by patients with cancer

1. *Knowledge of the diagnosis*
   - inadequacy of information
   - uncertainty about prognosis
   - guilt about causality
   - stigma of cancer
   - fear of a painful and undignified death
   - worries about reaction of family and friends

2. *Treatment side effects*
   - Surgery is often mutilating and can cause:
     body image problems
     loss of physical function
     loss of sexual function
   - Radiotherapy can cause:
     nausea and vomiting
     lethargy
     skin irritation
     anxiety and depression
   - Chemotherapy can cause:
     (hormonal or cytotoxic)
     nausea and vomiting
     alopecia
     mouth ulcers
     leucopenia
     cardiotoxicity
     hirsutism or feminization
     hot flushes

Inadequacy of Information

There is plenty of evidence to show that patients suffer considerable stress and anxiety as a consequence of receiving inadequate information from their doctors (Davis and Fallowfield 1991). Although the number of doctors who deliberately withhold the diagnosis of cancer from their patients has declined in this country over the past decade, many still withhold very important information about diagnostic tests, necessary treatment and commonly experienced side effects. They do so on the basis that such discussions will merely increase anxiety and depression or encourage patients to decline treatment. Such naive frameworks can be disputed both theoretically and empirically (Ley 1988). Furthermore, it has been shown that doctors are not very good at judging how much information their patients desire, e.g. Waitzkin (1984) found that doctors underestimated the patient's informational needs in 65% of 336 consultations.

Uncertainty

Coping with the uncertainty is one of the most psychologically noxious experiences of patients prior to diagnosis and many express relief when the diagnosis of cancer is confirmed. A good example of this can be seen in the following quotation taken from an interview with a patient with breast cancer.

> When he said 'the tests show it's cancer' I was actually quite relieved. It might sound silly, but at last someone had told me and I could stop worrying about what it might be. I couldn't wait to have the operation and start living again. I slept for the first time in two weeks that night.
>
> (Fallowfield 1991a)

The importance to good adjustment of adequate information at the time of diagnosis cannot be stressed strongly enough. Although ambiguity and evasion may appear to convey some short-term benefits they deny patients and their relatives an opportunity to accept and adapt successfully to the diagnosis and forthcoming treatment. The importance of accurate information about probable scarring following surgery is discussed later under body image, but one further point to consider is the effect that insufficient information can have on the doctor–patient relationship. The short-term benefits are that the doctor can avoid a potentially difficult and emotionally stressful consultation and the patient who may feel quite well after initial treatment may be able to minimize the seriousness of the disease. Indeed, there is some evidence that, as with coronary heart disease, in the absence of symptoms or signs of the disease patients with malignant melanoma tend to minimize its seriousness (Holland 1989). Most work done to date suggests that patients with malignant melanoma react to the diagnosis with initial distress followed by a positive outlook towards treatment, family, friends and life in general (Longman and Graham 1986). There is little doubt that the manner in which the diagnosis is conveyed affects psychological adjustment. Holland discusses the way in which uncertainty promotes anxiety and suggests that the major psychological problem experienced by patients following the diagnosis of melanoma is the sense of being a "walking time bomb". Unfortunately, if things do go wrong and issues such as the potential for metastatic spread have not been aired, the trust that the patient places in the clinician may have been irreparably compromised. The doctor who misleads patients with false reassurance at the outset when diagnosis and treatment is discussed will have difficulty later in convincing the patient with disseminated disease that their pain will be controlled or that they will not die a lonely, undignified death.

Prognosis

Unlike many cancer sites, clinicians using a combination of clinical and histological factors can usually provide patients who have malignant melanoma with useful prognostic information. For example, histopathological indicators may provide good estimates of disease progression and outcome. It is actually unusual for patients to ask how long they have left to live (Hogbin and Fallowfield 1989), although many do want some general estimates, such as weeks rather than months or months rather than years. Handing out an exact prophecy as to the likely course of the disease is akin to issuing the individual with a death sentence and should be avoided. If the doctor is wrong, the relatives may be triumphant about the patient exceeding the time "given" by the doctor or very angry if it proves shorter than predicted. Giving general information about prognosis, however, allows patients and their relatives to deal with "unfinished business" such as taking the much dreamed about trip somewhere or initiating reconciliations and resolving long-standing family feuds.

Guilt About Causality

It is not unusual for patients with cancer to feel that their disease is some sort of punishment or divine retribution for real or imagined improprieties. Most of us subscribe to an implicit faith in a "just-world"; thus the victims of cancer may sometimes feel blamed by others for having "caused" their own illness (Lerner and Miller 1978). Although this is seen primarily in those cancers where a direct causal link between behaviour and the disease has been established, such as smoking and lung cancer, this feeling of guilt and personal responsibility can occur in individuals with cancer at any site. An understanding of a patient's underlying beliefs about the causal factors for his or her melanoma may prove to be an important aspect of counselling. An interesting study by Kroode et al. (1989) compared causal attributions of cancer patients with those of patients with cardiac problems. The major finding of the study was that cardiac patients looked in their past histories for causes that correlated with medical opinion whereas cancer patients attributed their malignancy to extremely personal idiosyncratic causes bearing little relationship to causal factors expressed by their doctors or even their relatives. Patients often need the help of a counsellor to express and ventilate their anger at the "unfairness" of getting cancer. The following extract from an interview with a man with stomach cancer provides a good illustration.

> I just keep on thinking Why me? What have I done to deserve this? I've always put in a good day's work, never claimed any benefit and I think I did my fair share with the kids when they were small. I've never gone off with other women and apart from the odd beer after football or to be sociable I haven't been a bad husband. She never went without because I'd spent all my pay packet. It just doesn't seem fair to me at all.

> (quoted from Fallowfield 1991b)

Without counselling support to express and ventilate anger and to find a means of accepting the random unfairness of cancer, such patients can become consumed with their "Why me?" thoughts. They may become depressed, socially withdrawn and resentful of the seemingly undeserving well world, all of which may also make them feel guilty, thus compounding the psychological burden.

Guilt About Outcome

There has been a considerable amount of publicity given to some of the alternative cancer therapies which promote the notion that individuals can combat cancer through various dietary and psychological means. Some of these therapies may increase the burden of guilt shouldered by patients. Not only do they encourage the view that patients must and can take responsibility for the outcome of their disease, but they also imply that dietary indiscretions, a faulty lifestyle or personality "caused" the cancer in the first place. Even if the hypothesis that personality factors and coping style do enhance survival (and I will discuss some of the evidence for that later), changing entrenched personality style may be difficult if not impossible. This leaves patients with the added stress of knowing that they might have caused the cancer and also its progression. Maguire (1989) quotes an especially poignant example of the distress this can cause in a middle-aged woman with cancer:

> It's bad enough having cancer and knowing that I could die before my time. But to be told that it is because I have Type C personality is no help at all. I am 55 years of age. There is no way I am going to change the kind of person I am now.

Undoubtedly, some patients gain a great deal from the feeling that they can assert some control over the course of their disease by making major lifestyle changes, but there are dangers other than patients assuming too much responsibility for a poor outcome. The primary source of help and support is the patient's own family and friends and a sudden change in personality from quiet introversion to over-assertiveness may well seriously undermine the dynamics of these important relationships at a crucial time. Counsellors may need to offer help and support to the family of a patient who is attempting major life changes as a result of cancer.

Fear of Dying

Although many diseases are as seriously life-threatening as cancer, malignancy is subjectively more terrifying to the majority of lay people. Many see cancer and death as synonymous and are very pessimistic about the mortality figures for cancer (Knopf 1974). Patients also fear that death will be intolerably and uncontrollably painful, and that they will suffer the indignity of loss of control of bodily functions. Abandonment by family and friends is another frequently expressed fear. As we shall see later in this chapter patients with malignant melanoma in particular often attempt to control their anxieties by repressing such fears. This may be a satisfactory coping strategy for some, but an opportunity to discuss fears and worries with someone capable of dealing with the powerful emotions such conversations may evoke should always be offered (Fallowfield 1990).

Treatment Side Effects

The physical side effects of chemotherapy and radiotherapy are well known. Many clinicians are less familiar with the psychological problems associated with these treatments. The impact of chemotherapy and radiotherapy has on quality of life of patients has been fully described elsewhere (Fallowfield, 1990), but it should be noted that significant numbers of patients develop anxiety and depression together with enervating fatigue following these treatments. Some may also develop conditioned responses such as anticipatory nausea and vomiting which need the help of a psychologist skilled in systematic desensitization and relaxation techniques.

Body Image Problems

As far as the emotional implications of scarring after surgery for malignant melanoma are concerned, Cassileth (1983) and her colleagues have shown the importance of adequate preoperative information. In study of 176 patients' perceptions of the cosmetic impact of melanoma resection, they found that those patients whose scar size had been anticipated accurately were significantly less distressed than those whose scars were larger than expected. Overall 70% of the men and 64% of the women felt that their scars were larger than they had been led to anticipate. There was an interesting sex difference in terms of scar visibility and distress, with men being more distressed by scars normally covered by clothing and women maximally distressed by visible scars. The study showed that patients were more concerned about indentation than scar length, were more distressed if inadequately prepared for size of the scar, and that primary closure rather than skin grafting conveyed important psychological benefits to patients. The authors concluded that "The most effective preventive intervention against psychological distress would appear to be improved physician-patient communication."

Psychiatric Morbidity

It is important for all those caring for patients with malignant melanoma to appreciate that virtually all patients will, at some stage of their illness, experience periods of anxiety, depression, social and sexual dysfunction. Although many will find means of coping with their difficulties, there is plenty of evidence that for a significant minority of patients the problems persist and remain severe and unremitting without help. Using a standardized psychiatric interview Derogatis et al. (1983) found that 44% of 215 newly diagnosed patients with cancer admitted to hospital had adjustment and mood disorders, of which anxiety and/or depression were predominant. Likewise, Bukberg et al. (1984) interviewed 62 patients and reported that depression was rated as severe in 24% of the sample, moderate in 18% and mild in a further 14% (compare these figures with the point prevalence of depression for the general population which is around 9%–20%, Boyd and Weissman 1981). Even experienced oncologists are often surprised by the high rates of affective disorder revealed by these studies and there are many reasons why much of the psychiatric morbidity is unrecognized and consequently goes untreated. Table 13.2 provides a summary of the myths that exist about the relative importance of discussing psychosocial problems with patients in comparison to treating the physical aspects of cancer. It is a sorry reflection of the state of medical education with its adherence to a biological rather than biopsychosocial

Table 13.2. Reasons for avoiding discussion of psychosocial concerns with patients

Myths	Reality
1. My patients will tell me if they feel depressed or anxious.	1. Patients will not volunteer such information unless encouraged to do so.
2. Depression and anxiety are "normal" consequences of having cancer, so there is nothing I can do about it.	2. They are common reactions to cancer that are readily amenable to treatment. Pain is "normal" following surgery, but no-one uses that as a reason for withholding analgesics.
3. It is more important that I get on with treating the cancer – emotional issues are not part of my responsibility.	3. Doctors feel more comfortable dealing with physical concerns. They feel emotionally vulnerable themselves when exploring psychosocial issues.
4. I am too busy to deal with emotional issues. I would if I had the time.	4. Medical education does not equip doctors very well with communication skills that permit them to be emphatic and open within a realistic time-frame.

model of medicine that many doctors know more about the characteristics of malignant tumour cells than they do about the unfortunate patient harbouring them. Even worse is the fact that, when the communication problems and counselling needs of patients are identified, doctors may feel ill-equipped to deal with them. Clinicians may then use a variety of distancing tactics or justifications for avoiding discussion of those issues so important to the satisfactory adjustment of their patients.

Personality and Malignant Melanoma

The past decade has seen increasing interest in the part that the interaction of psychological and biological variables may play in both the expression of melanoma and subsequent survival (Rogentine et al. 1979; Temoshok 1985). Many patients with malignant melanoma exhibit the so-called Type C personality (Temoshok and Fox 1984) which is characterized primarily by "emotional containment". Individuals with Type C do not appear to be able to express emotion very easily, especially anger. They tend to be co-operative, unassertive, self-sacrificing people who are very accepting or compliant with external authorities. Such characteristics are the polar opposite of Type A personality which has been shown to be prevalent among people who later develop heart disease (Rosenman et al. 1964). An interesting study showing the personality differences betweeen these different disease groups was reported by Kneier and Temoshok (1984). They measured the electrodermal activity of 20 patients with melanoma, 20 with cardiovascular disease and 20 controls who were all shown 50 anxiety provoking statements which they were asked to rate on a scale 0–10 for how much the statement "bothered me". Results showed the melanoma patients to be significantly more repressed than the other two groups on both self-report and physiological measures. This work may have important implications for the outcome of malignant melanoma and means of influencing it through various cognitive interventions. Some recent research into the psychosocial factors influencing disease progression has shown that emotional expression of sadness and anger is positively correlated with tumour-specific host–response factors and negatively correlated with mitotic rate (Temoshok 1985). Some psychotherapeutic approaches are designed to facilitate the constructive expression of anger (Moorey and Greer 1989), but evidence that this might alter behaviour sufficiently to affect outcome is equivocal. The whole area of psychoneuroimmunology is contentious, but there is evidence that patients with thicker, more invasive tumours are less narcissistic and less histrionic and more likely to be passive, appeasing and helpless than active, impatient and controlling. They also have a strong external locus of control placing faith in God and/or doctors. This association between Type C coping style and unfavourable prognostic indices could well be behaviourally mediated; in other words, Type C individuals may be less likely to seek medical attention. Another hypothesis could be that Type C features are associated with various biological responses which may enhance tumour development and/or depress the immune response.

Psychosocial Factors and Delay

Considerable efforts have been made to inform the public about the hazards of sun-worship and to warn particularly fair-skinned individuals to be vigilant about any changes in pigmented moles or freckles. Despite this increased awareness of the risk factors and need to seek medical advice about suspicious lesions, approximately 30% of melanoma patients already have evidence of metastatic disease, suggesting that there has been a significant time lapse between recognition of the lesion and presentation to a physician. As the length of delay is significantly associated with unfavourable prognostic indicators, it is important to understand the modifying behavioural factors related to delay.

An impressive series of studies (Temoshok et al. 1984; Temoshok 1985) has shown that patient delay in reporting the melanoma emerged as the most significant variable predicting tumour thickness. The factors relating to longer delays are summarized in Table 13.3. The fact that studies have shown an increase in delay in patients with back lesions in comparison to other sites highlights the way in which denial operates most effectively in individuals with lesions in less visibly accessible places. It is easier to deny or forget about the existence of a lesion on the back than it would be for one on the face or hand, for example. Increasing public education about the need to report suspicious lesions early should perhaps include encouragement to tell one's friends and family about

Table 13.3. Factors related to delay in seeking medical attention (Temoshok 1985)

Site of lesion (back longer than other sites)
Less previous knowledge of melanoma
Less understanding of treatment
Less minimization of its seriousness

changes in pigmentation of sites that they are unlikely to monitor carefully themselves.

Other factors contributing to delay, such as less knowledge and understanding of melanoma and treatment, are easily understood, but the fact that delay is correlated with less minimization of seriousness needs explanation. It seems a counterintuitive finding, but patients who are able to minimize the seriousness of their condition may seek out medical advice sooner, as they may experience less anxiety and fear about diagnosis or its treatment.

Psychological Aftercare

So how can doctors be helped to provide better psychological aftercare for their patients with malignant melanoma? There are a number of good communication and counselling skills training courses being organized for postgraduate medical staff that go some way to rectify the inadequate training that most doctors have recieved in these areas. Unfortunately, this is not a viable option for everyone. At the very least, clinicians should be aware of the characteristics (Table 13.4) of those patients most likely to experience adjustment difficulties and who may be most in need of counselling intervention. Some GPs now employ professional counsellors within their practices, who may be able to offer the "at risk" patients help with the adoption of the most adaptive and effective coping strategies. Other patients may live in the vicinity of a hospital which has the services of an oncology counsellor or a liaison psychiatrist who specializes in psychotherapy for oncology patients. It is important to recognize that counselling is a professional skill that requires quite lengthy training and supervision. All too often the term is used rather loosely to describe anything from general advice giving, to tea, sympathy and a shoulder to cry on (Fallowfield 1988). Although these approaches might provide patients with some temporary short-term comfort they are unlikely to bring about the sorts of adaptive coping strategies necessary to help a distressed patient come to terms with their illness. Unfortunately, many of the people employed to counsel have received insufficient training to help patients effectively (Fallowfield 1991c).

There are some other fairly basic means of improving the psychological care of patients with malignant melanoma (Table 13.5). These include the importance of

Table 13.4. Characteristics of patients most likely to experience poor coping and adjustment

Patients who have:
- received poor information about illness and treatment
- a view of their doctors as unhelpful
- a history of alcohol or drug abuse
- a previous psychiatric history
- a pessimistic, helpless, hopeless outlook
- inflexible, rigid coping strategies
- inadequate social support, or who perceive social support to be inadequate
- a history of recent noxious life events, especially losses

Table 13.5. Ways of improving counselling and aftercare of patients with malignant melanoma

---

- Make sure that patients are properly informed about their illness and treatment
- Give patients an opportunity to discuss emotional problems, not just physical
- Be aware of characteristics of patients most at risk of developing serious psychiatric morbidity
- Refer patients identified as suffering from adjustment disorders to appropriately trained counsellors or psychotherapists
- Involve, inform and support the person identified by the patient as their primary social supporter

---

ensuring that patients and their relatives are well-informed about the likely course of their disease and the implications of different treatments. Poor communication between nursing, radiotherapy and medical staff in hospitals often means that essential discussions about treatment and side effects are not mentioned to the patient as everyone assumes that someone else has raised the issues. This problem may become magnified by communication failures between the hospital and the patient's GP.

Patients need an opportunity to discuss the emotional problems that their disease and treatment may provoke. This may require considerable skill as individuals with malignant melanoma tend to have somewhat repressed personality profiles and may minimize problems in an attempt to alleviate anxiety. If this coping strategy is not successful then these patients need careful counselling designed to facilitate the expression of negative emotions and to encourage the adoption of more appropriate, realistic means of coping.

Being aware of the characteristics of those patients most at risk of developing serious psychiatric morbidity may allow the clinician to refer patients at an early stage to appropriately trained oncology counsellors.

Finally, cancer is never just a problem for the affected individual. It has a major impact on the lives of family and friends. They too need help and support, especially as it is they who will have to provide the patient with support over the course of the disease, whatever the outcome.

References

Boyd JH, Weissman MM (1981) Epidemiology of affective disorders. A re-examination and future direction. Arch Gen Psychiatry 38:1039–1046

Bukberg J, Penman D, Holland JC (1984) Depression in hospitalised cancer patients. Psychosom Med 46:199–212

Cassileth BR, Lusk EJ, Tenaglia AN (1983) Patients' perceptions of the cosmetic impact of melanoma resection. Plas Reconstr Surg 71:73–75

Davis H, Fallowfield LJ (eds.) (1991) Counselling and communication in health care. Wiley, Chichester

Derogatis LR, Morrow GR, Fetting J et al. (1983) The prevalence of psychiatric disorders among cancer patients. JAMA 249:751–757

Fallowfield LJ (1988) Counselling for patients with cancer. Br Med J 297:727–728

Fallowfield LJ (1990) The quality of life: the missing measurement in health care. Souvenir Press, London

Fallowfield LJ (1991a) Breast cancer. Routledge, London

Fallowfield LJ (1991b) In: Davis H, Fallowfield LJ (eds.) Counselling and communication in health care. Wiley, Chichester, p 260

Fallowfield LJ (1991c) Counselling and communication in oncology. Br J Cancer 63:481–482

Hogbin B, Fallowfield LJ (1989) Getting it taped: the "bad news" consultation with cancer patients. Br J Hosp Med 41:330–333

Holland JC (1989) Skin cancer and melanoma. In: Holland JC, Rowland JH (eds.) Handbook of psychooncology. Psychological care of the patient with cancer. Oxford University Press, New York

Klein E, Burgess GH, Helm F (1973) Neoplasms of the skin. In: Holland F, Frei E (eds.) Cancer medicine. Lea & Febiger, Philadelphia

Kneier AW, Temoshok L (1984) Repressive coping reactions in patients with malignant melanoma as compared to cardiovascular disease patients. J Psychosom Res 28(2):14–155

Kroode H, Oosterwijk M, Steverink N (1989) Three conflicts as a result of causal attributions. Soc Sci Med 28:93–97

Knopf A (1974) Cancer: changes in opinion after 7 years of public education in Lancaster. Manchester Regional Committee on Cancer, Manchester

Lerner MJ, Miller DT (1978) Just world research and the attribution process: looking back and ahead. Psychol Bull 85:1030–1051

Ley P (1988) Communicating with patients: improving communication satisfaction and compliance. Croom Helm, London

Longman AJ, Graham KY (1986) Living with melanoma: content analysis of interviews. Oncol Nurs Forum 13(4):58–64

Maguire P (1989) Breast conservation versus mastectomy: psychological considerations. Semin Surg Oncol 5:137–144

Moorey S, Greer S (1989) Psychological therapy for patients with cancer. Heinemann, Oxford

Rogentine GN, Van Kammen DF, Fox BH et al. (1979) Psychological factors in the prognosis of malignant melanoma. Psychosom Med 41:647–658

Rosenman R, Friedman M, Straus R et al. (1964) A predictive study of coronary heart disease. JAMA 189:15–26

Temoshok L (1985) Biopsychosocial studies on cutaneous malignant melanoma: psychosocial factors associated with prognostic indicators, progression, psychophysiology and tumour–host response. Soc Sci Med 20:833–840

Temoshok L, Fox B (1984) Coping styles and other psychosocial factors related to medical status and prognosis in patients with cutaneous malignant melanoma. In: Fox B, Newberry B (eds.) Impact of psychoendocrine systems in cancer and immunity. Hogrefe, Toronto

Temoshok L, Di Clemente RJ, Sweed DM et al. (1984) Factors related to patient delay in seeking medical attention for cutaneous malignant melanoma. Cancer 54:3048–3053

Waitzkin H (1984) Doctor–patient communication: Implications of social scientific research. JAMA 252:2441–2446

Subject Index